Beyond AA

In the Front Door, Then out the Back Door...
30 Years of AA & ADD to a life of Unity (& ADD).

Howard Casanova

©**Copyright 2014** Howard Casanova
Casanova: *Beyond AA*
All rights reserved.

ISBN: 1503159442
ISBN 13: 9781503159440
Library of Congress Control Number: 2014920299
LCCN Imprint Name:

DISCLAIMER

All of the opinions given are the author's and are as accurate as he could make them. Also, out of respect for the anonymity factor of AA, he has written this book under a pseudonym.

Preface

If you are presently attending AA and are happy with the results, you do not need to read further, because...

The purpose of this book is an attempt to answer the question: "Do you believe you are either: an alcoholic/addict who needs weekly recovery meetings *for the rest of your life* or simply an abuser who needs to clean up his or her act?"

If you are still wrestling with that, read on.

This topic and its conclusions came out of a life-changing episode of "perfect storm" dimensions. Three years ago, as a sixty-five-year-old man, I had seen my life *as I had known i*t go suddenly "off course," and to cope with this, I began journaling. My career had crashed, my marriage of twenty-seven years had ended suddenly, and I was nearly broke.

One of the first things I discovered on this trip was how little my three decades of attendance in Alcoholics Anonymous (AA), have now influenced this recovery I desperately had to achieve.

AA was no longer the safe harbor it had been for me—no longer the floatation device or life preserver tossed to a victim who had washed overboard. Instead, it offered virtually no solutions at all—because I had finally outgrown it—and you're not supposed to do that.

I still followed the principles (see axioms after the last chapter) of "the program," but the life solutions that AA had offered me no longer applied. I no longer needed to recover from alcohol and drug abuse; I just needed to live or die and to decide which one to do. I chose to live, tacked, and changed course. By continuing my struggle, I persevered and ultimately grew from this calamity. Along the way, the diary I had started to help myself cope became this story of discovery and of a new direction for a life that was very much streaming toward a crash on rocky shoals.

I developed insights into, as AA puts it in their publication, Alcoholics Anonymous, hereafter known as; the Big Book, on p.58; "what we used to be like, what happened and what we are like now."

AA and I had grown up together. It had changed from the evangelical religious movement it had started life as, to the treatment-industry aftercare program it is today. I, with AA's guidance, had become a responsible adult.

And then, one day, we no longer needed each other.

CONTENTS

Introduction
    "Gimme Some Old-Time Religion…"...................8

Chapter 1
    An Old-Time AA Meeting.....................11

Chapter 2
    A Homicidal Drunk-a-Log.....................14

Chapter 3
    What Changed Then—AA or Me?...................18

Chapter 4
    A Troubled Youth.....................24

Chapter 5
    Adulthood, More Trouble.....................32

Chapter 6
    Beverly Hills's AA in Minnesota.....................36

Chapter 7
    What I Found AA to Be Like, at First...............40

Chapter 8
    When AA Changed Forever.....................43

Chapter 9
    The AA Cure.....................49

Chapter 10
    Starting Over Again.....................55

Chapter 11
    Sobriety Gone, Then Found Again.....................57

Chapter 12
    A New Start, with Ladies Too.....................62

Chapter 13
    Sailing Through Thirty Years of AA
    and Changes.....................64

Chapter 14
    Out the Back Door of AA.....................71

Chapter 15
    My Perfect Storm 80
Chapter 16
    Is AA the Only Way? 88
Chapter 17
    Why Bother to Write This Book? 93
Chapter 18
    In Defense of AA, but also of the 90+ Percent
    Who Cannot, Will Not Fit-in There 95
Chapter 19
    AA and Emotional Breakdowns 102
Chapter 20
    Where Did This Train Go "Off the Tracks"? .104
Chapter 21
    Summary 109
My Axioms 119
The Beer/Wine Diet 122

Introduction
"Gimme Some Old-Time Religion…"

For thirty-five years, I, a former pothead, regularly attended AA meetings. This is the story of what I witnessed of the recovery industry and the changes it brought to the AA meetings and why I finally had to outgrow the organization.

Consider this: fewer than one in ten of those attending AA are regulars—what I came to call the "true believers" who benefit from the teaching and sharing done in meetings.

This explains why most attendees of AA meetings will never return after their first visit(s), but (stay with me here), the continual new referrals who keep showing up keep the place looking full. I've come to call this phenomenon the "revolving door."

Voluminous research has been done on this topic.

An Internet search for "results of AA recovery" might cause some dismay among AA supporters.

For instance, one source, Dr. Stanton Peele, PhD, claimed in a 1998 article in *The Sciences, p.17 – 21,* that; "the most widely used 12 step treatment is the least effective. Brief intervention in motivational therapy is more successful"![1]

Dr. Lance Dodes sees a big problem with 12 step programs. The psychiatrist has spent more than 20 years studying and treating addiction. His latest book on the subject is *The Sober Truth: Debunking the Bad Science Behind 12-Step Programs and the Rehab Industry. He gives AA no better than a* **5-10 percent** *recovery rate and further claims the 90 percent failure rate is harmful to the recovering person.*[2]

Another source—Professor George Vaillant of Harvard University, who just happened at the time to be a member of the AA World Services Board of Trustees—came to a similar conclusion when he participated in the 1983 *Cambridge Somerville Program for Alcohol Rehabilitation* (CASPAR) Study.[3] This study followed the results of a twenty-four-hour walk-in service with medical treatment for detoxing and found that out of more than 1000 inpatient and 20,000 outpatient visits in one year, only 2500 were treated for detoxification!

Achieving long-term sobriety usually involves (1) a less harmful, substitute dependency; (2) new relationships; (3) sources of inspiration and hope; and (4) experiencing negative consequences of drinking.[3]

Vaillant argues that AA and other similar groups effectively harness the above four factors of healing and that many alcoholics achieve sobriety through AA attendance. However, he also notes that the "effectiveness of AA has not been adequately assessed"[63] and that **direct evidence for the efficacy of AA… remains as elusive as ever.**[64] For example, if an alcoholic achieves sobriety during AA attendance, **who is to say if AA helped or if he merely went to AA when he was ready to heal?**[9][65]

In the Clinic sample, 48% of the 29 alcoholics who achieved sobriety eventually attended 300 or more AA meetings,[66] and AA attendance was associated with good outcomes in patients who otherwise would have been predicted not to remit.[67] In the Core City sample the more severe alcoholics attended AA, possibly because all other avenues had failed—after all, **AA meetings are rarely attended for hedonistic reasons.**[68] The implication from all three samples was simply that **many**, not most, alcoholics find help through AA.[69]

And remember, this guy was one of AA's friends!

Speaking of AA's friends when the Big Book of AA, *Alcoholics Anonymous,* was published, the October 1939 volume of the <u>Journal of the American Medical Association</u> (JAMA)[4] in a book review, called the book **"A curious combination of organizing propaganda and religious exhortation…in no sense a scientific book. Strongly reminiscent of Dale Carnegie and of the Buchman (Oxford) movement."**

In the seventy-five years since, JAMA has never retracted this statement!

Under my watch, a "new" AA came to be, and the changes I'll share with you were dramatic. To protect the anonymity of those who were part of this discovery, names of all individuals and names and stated locations of the AA clubs are fictitious. Any resemblance to actual persons or existing facilities is coincidental and unintentional.

"Some old-time religion is good enough for me."

Chapter 1
An Old-Time AA Meeting

1975. The bright, full moon did nothing to ease the chill of the northeast wind blowing down University Boulevard on this frigid February evening. It was only 5:30 p.m., and already this northern city was in full nightfall. The bright moonlight, however, illuminated the details of the building I was seeking. The brick walls on the downtown AA club were a pale shade of grime thanks to more than eight decades on a busy urban thoroughfare. The faded sign on the upper wall indicated that the building had formerly housed a business that sold and serviced typewriters and copy machines. Never having been here before, I found this experience was very much unlike going to my home AA group in a nice, clean suburban church basement. This downtown AA club was not a nice place at all.

Pungent, sinus-burning nicotine tar odors wafted off the yellow-stained walls, ceilings, floors, and everything else. That included unwashed bodies—some of the locals here still slept under bridges in cardboard boxes and alleyways. They too were regulars at these AA meetings finding free coffee, cookies, shelter, and, today, maybe sobriety.

A couple of volunteers nodded a greeting at me inside the lobby. They would've offered help if asked; more likely, though, they assumed any visitor knew why he was there. Everything else you needed to know was on the walls. Posted were mimeographed, typed lists of meeting rooms numbered with days and times of the various squads, including some for nonsmokers! Women's AA and, also Al-Anon meetings were posted also, as well as more yellowed signs and slogans:

"My worst day sober is better than my best day drinking."

"Let go and let God."

"K. I. S. S. Keep it simple, stupid."

The walls also held a framed pair of eulogies (complete with portrait photos) of the founders of AA in 1935—Dr. Bob S (Smith) and Bill W (Wilson)—last names withheld because of their anonymity, though this was not necessary any longer because *they've both been dead for decades!*

There were, too, large posters of the "12 Steps" and the "12 Traditions" of AA and smaller ones announcing club hours and general rules of conduct, one of which was *not yet* no smoking. For most, this would not seem to be a fun place unless you found their secret elixir, as many others and I had!

This elixir was the magic-like buzz you rather quickly absorbed from a banquet of sugar-loaded, strong coffee, handfuls of cookies, and tobacco-smoke-induced nicotine—a triple shot, if there ever was one. Almost all members of early AA meetings sobered up in this way!

Some serious multitasking was going on in here: drink the coffee, eat the snacks, smoke while managing the ashes, listen, and participate (stand up, sit down, raise your hand, etc.), while not spilling or burning anything! All this while seated in lumpy, worn, nicotine-marinated couches and chairs.

I got a cup, went in, and found a seat. A dozen or so men and a few women were there, mostly middle-aged or older. Many were poorly dressed. A few shirts and ties, though the women were generally not fixed up.

The room already held a gray haze. Many smoked cigars or pipes, too, as they reported on their sobriety. By the end of the meeting, which lasted at least an hour, you could not see across the room. The smoke caused eyes to burn. An exhaust fan drew out some of the fog, barely. Going no smoking later on was one of the good changes to AA.

At least they weren't drinking alcohol, too, I thought—at least, most weren't.

I learned later how much like an old-time original AA meeting this was. This group was one of the few AA clubs that still followed a church-auditorium-style format in which a squad leader called a speaker up before an audience of sober attendees, as opposed to the "group therapy" format so popular today because of the treatment centers. Some of these members were old enough to have been there from AA's earliest beginning.

The squad leader called the meeting to order, the Serenity Prayer was announced, and everyone stood and recited:
> "God grant me the serenity to accept the things I cannot change, the courage to change the things I can, and the wisdom to know the difference. Amen."

The leader then took care of club business and read the announcements. Today's meeting would be of a "tell your personal story" format. We went around the room with personal declaration-introductions:
"My name is Howard, and I'm an alcoholic," followed by "Hi, Howard," and so on.

Note: Of the two dozen plus men and women in this mid-1970 meeting, not one of them would claim to be a drug addict or chemically dependent. They were all simply "drunks or alcoholics." In today's AA climate, this would not be possible; most now will claim to be "chemically dependent."

Chapter 2
A Homicidal Drunk-a-Log

1975. The squad leader introduced the only speaker for the night: a man named Lefty B., tall and slightly stooped, gaunt with a whisker stubble and longish, graying hair, dark eyes, and pale complexion. He looked the part, still wearing a gray industrial uniform with black work shoes; I had observed him upon our entering together.

"My name is Lefty, and I'm an alcoholic."

"Hi, Lefty."

"By the grace of God and the fellowship of Alcoholics Anonymous, I have not had a drink of alcohol for eleven years, six months, and twenty-three days."

Applause.

"I must tell you, becoming a member of AA was never a part of any plans I'd had for my life, and I never thought I'd be giving my story to any kind of a group!"

He went on.

"About ten years ago, I had been in the army infantry and my tour was up, so I mustered out. I admit to drinking some in the army, sometimes too much, and even ended up in the brig. Getting home, I found work as a construction laborer. A while later, I married my girlfriend and we settled down."

He paused to sip his still-steaming coffee, as did everyone else.

A loud "slurp" filled the room.

"Shortly after this," he said, *"two guys I wish now hadn't found me dropped in at my home to invite me out for some beers. My new bride was not happy about this, but she didn't interfere."*

He paused to scan the room again.

"I admit I should not have gone with these guys, knowing probably no good could come of it. We went to a local saloon, where, after probably more than a few drinks, somebody got the foolish idea it would be fun to rob a gas station, just for 'kicks.' The one down the block, which was closed for the night. It had pretty big windows kind of hidden in the back wall."

He/we sip more coffee.

*"Easy money, we thought. What we did not think about, and nobody brought up, was how really stupid this was, **before** we actually went ahead with it."*

Laughter.

"We forced open the rear shop window and all three of us crawled into the building. However, without our realizing it, the cops had been alerted by the garage silent alarm, while we were busy looking for money and other things to steal. We didn't hear them arrive. They had silently crept into the front door with their passkey. Suddenly the lights were thrown on—I felt my blood turn to ice water when one of the cops shouted at us, 'Everyone freeze and lie down on the floor!'"

The next place where Lefty B. lay down was in a jail cell on a hard steel cot with no pillow.

"The next day in court, since my only prior had been a juvenile record for mischief, the judge gave me a ninety-day jail sentence plus probation for a year."

This should've been the end of a stupid prank and maybe a valuable life experience. He went on.

"My wife, no children yet, agreed to stay with me through this if I'd clean up my act. I was relieved. It could've been worse."

Many of the men listening to him tonight had had similar adventures of inebriation, similar, at least, until he got to the rest of his story.

"Three months went by. I served my time and was released on probation, a condition of which was no drinking, but what I hadn't yet taken into account about myself was that I was prone to suffer a condition known as blackouts."

He continued.

"I guess this is like knowing you're a diabetic or you have a serious allergy. A person needs to be responsible and manage these things," he said. *"I never tried to do this. I would guzzle, not sip, my drinks, and this then would result in a blackout. I've since learned a diabetic will suffer a similar fate from an excessive sugar intake.*

"To anyone watching me during these periods, I would appear to be acting normally—tipsy, but otherwise seemingly OK. In actuality, I had no idea what I was doing, and afterward had no recall of what I did do during the episode."

More coffee, and a puff on a cigarette. He rubbed his eyes with a sleeve. The smoke was getting to him too.

"So, when I awoke again in a jail cell with a terrible hangover one morning, I had no idea why I was there. Obviously, I suspected drinking had something to do with it."

It seems he had done the "blackout" thing again the night before, but he didn't know about this yet.

He would soon find out.

"We inmates were manacled to a chain by a sheriff's deputy holding the other nine or ten jailed prisoners: whites, blacks, Latinos—human trash and citizens alike—some of us still well-buzzed from the night before. All of us surly, as we were marched into the adjacent city hall and courtroom, where we would hear the charges against us."

He paused again for a drink of his coffee and to snuff out his smoldering cigarette butt.

"When my turn was called, I stepped up before this pissed-off looking judge as the charges were read out to the courtroom by the bailiff.

"I just about shit my pants when I heard mine. If I hadn't grabbed the court-rail before me, I would have collapsed onto the floor. I learned I had been drinking the night before and then driving drunk, too. Early morning at daybreak, I'd lost control of my car, which jumped the street curbing, then ran down a small child being taken to school by his mother and then crashed the car into a tree."

He went on in a now-quaking voice.

"The cops arrived to find the mother unconscious and seriously injured. The child was dead at the scene; they found me passed out in the wreckage."

The room was silent. I had never heard such a devastating, self-condemning story. I didn't know whether to hate Lefty, pity him, or both. Lefty went on:

"I was sentenced to ten years of hard-time in the state prison; my wife did leave me this time, changed her name, and has disappeared from my life. In prison, I found God and AA in the same meeting, and it saved my life. I was released last year and have been going to meetings here ever since."

Lefty then closed with a thank-you and was given a small round of applause from the rest of the group. The squad leader closed the meeting with the Lord's Prayer. We then all filed out to repair to the lunchroom in the rear of the building for more coffee, smoking, and visiting. Where everyone was usually talkative and upbeat after a meeting, not today—solemnity pervaded this group. We would never forget Lefty's story.

I had learned a lesson about forgiveness from it too. Over the years, I befriended Lefty, and after more than three decades, communicate with him on Facebook and find him to still be a deeply spiritual person who seems to have found peace in his life. He still attends AA and sponsors a few fortunate men.

In attending more meetings at this club, I heard stories of failure and redemption from other drunks; none would ever eclipse Lefty's though. Many were similar because these drunks discovered—almost accidentally—that they could not guzzle or binge-drink alcohol without suffering severe consequences.

As I look back over those years, I recall that also among this group were the true hard-core alcoholics early AA had cared for: the chronic alcoholics who would lose control if they had more than a couple of drinks. To these unfortunates, their addiction is akin to an addiction to heroin, and, according to some, likely worse.

Chapter 3
What Changed Then—AA or Me?

2014. This book describes my thirty-five-year journey within, then finally out of, AA. Pertinent question here: "Why would an admitted pothead join and stay in AA for all of those years?" The answer, I suspect, is that my untreated ADD (attention deficit disorder) had a lot to do with it.

AA took me in and allowed me to stay as long as I liked. I also met a lot of other closet-ADD sufferers there, too. The program and its twelve steps gave us all a guide to live by, helping us with our distresses, and we actually learned to function better in our daily lives.

Three years ago. I resigned from my local AA club because I could not break their ultimate pledge, which is to never return to drinking beverage alcohol, and yet still be considered an active AA member. AA maintains you are either in or you're out, and there is no graduation program here.

One day, following a long period of questioning myself about this decision, I decided for my own good reasons that I could finally manage moderate drinking. I had recently turned sixty-five, and, not surprisingly, had a "bucket list" of things I wanted to do before my time was up!

After twenty-nine years of practicing abstinence, you can believe having a beer or a glass of wine "whenever I wanted to" was near the top of the list! Then, one March evening, my then-wife, Susie, came home and announced to me, "I have something to tell you."

As far as I knew up to this point, she'd had one more year of sobriety than I had.

She continued, "I have been drinking alcohol since last August. Are you angry?" Hell no, I wasn't angry. I only wanted to know if she was all right. I had suspected she hadn't been going to AA meetings during this time (I hadn't been).

"Yes, I'm doing fine with it," she announced.

And so after pouring each other a celebratory glass of wine, I had my first drink of beverage alcohol in more than twenty-nine years! It was a Cabernet. I swished it around in my mouth as instructed and swallowed; it was delicious, even better than I'd remembered. I sniffed the next sip before drinking it; it was even more delicious than the first. We talked late into the evening on only two glasses of wine; the alcohol definitely relaxed us both so the conversation seemed to flow.

We chattered on about the huge change this represented to us both: after a lifetime of abstinence and AA attendance, all had changed a full 180 degrees. We both understood, more than most, how self-control and moderation-management of alcohol consumption would become of paramount importance.

And so after a stretch of twenty-nine years, and thirty-five years total of abstinence, I had decided to quit AA again—quit going to meetings and going out to the weekly dinner after-the-meeting, quit going to sober parties, quit sponsoring newcomers, quit taking the daily pledge, etc. Twenty-nine years, and suddenly everything changes!

So, by all of these actions, I have given up the life of an active member of AA. It feels funny to say this now after having been one for so long a time. The AA philosophy adamantly says you should not be able to do this—to drink successfully!

A huge part of the AA mantra is that a true alcoholic cannot tolerate even the first drink of alcohol.

Well, evidently a lot (as many as half, some studies say) of former AA members have done so too, I discovered. Since starting to drink again, I've met many such former members who all say pretty much the same thing: they tried AA, got tired of various aspects of it, quit it, and now today they are doing fine. Some are socially drinking too.

My daughter-in-law, who had only known me during my last twenty years of abstinence, when I was still preaching the AA gospel, was deeply chagrined and skeptical at first when I announced I had finally quit all that.

Then, recently, at a holiday gathering where beer and wine were being served, she told me in front of all of the family she'd accepted what I'd done. "Howard, even though you are sixty-five years old now, you act like you have just turned twenty-one, trying these new wines and drinks like it's your first time!" Exactly how it felt to me too.

I have now chosen to sit at the "other" adults' table, as it were, and I've found to my pleasure I am well accepted. This feels splendid, and I'm quite sure it will continue to, just so long as I uphold my end of the deal, which is to not abuse the privilege!

As of this writing, it has been more than three years since I've become a social drinker, primarily of wine and beer. And yet AA always insists in its teachings, which are read and preached at most meetings, that if you, as an alcoholic try to manage your drinking, you will eventually drink uncontrollably and—very likely—die from it.

Question: Does this not assume then that you truly must be a chronic alcoholic of the type the original AA was trying to treat? And not the court-ordered or treatment-center-referred, chemically dependent type of person that AA mostly serves today, both alcoholics and addicts included?

I have concluded that in my own case, I was a chronic pot (marijuana) smoker but not a heavy drinker. Did I ever abuse alcohol? Yes. But, did I ever really achieve a "seemingly hopeless state of mind and body," as the founders described it in the book of Alcoholics Anonymous? Not really. Does one actually ever get cured of this condition?

AA says emphatically no!

But many do recover—and go on to live successful lives. Some even go so far as to become socially drinking adults. And they do it without the help of AA or NA (Narcotics Anonymous) or any other support groups or programs, as I have been doing for over three years—so far.

On the other hand, it seems that the good old law "actions have consequences" eventually does dictate that certain types of users cannot abuse alcohol or any other chemicals without suffering a real backlash.

Examples of adverse consequences include divorce, breakups, family crisis, job-loss, fights, physical and emotional damage, arrests, etc. Each wields its own painful lesson to encourage self-control or the outright abstinence of the use of alcohol or recreational drugs.

This is not, as the AA program preaches, "Exclusively" the threat of having a disease! For example, you probably weren't a diseased driver when you drove a car into a tree, but you certainly were driving drunk. Rather than worrying about disease, we should be learning from our mistakes. For example, consider a child who cries, "It really hurts when I do that."

Reply: "Then don't do that anymore."

Simple.

Or, further imagine that you go out one day to get fitted for a new suit. When the sales clerk says, "Let's measure you for a fit," you say, "No thanks, just give me the one-size-fits-all suit this time."

Are you kidding?

Let's try one more analogy to help understand the AA/treatment industry way of thinking:

You've moved into a new town. It is a small city and quite remote. You soon find that the only medical facility there of any kind is the exclusive cancer-treatment hospital and clinic.

One day, you fall and break your arm. You then must go to the only medical facility, which is the cancer center. A doctor looks at you and immediately prescribes chemotherapy for your broken arm.

Fantastic?

Not in the world of treatment centers and AA. One diagnosis fits all here! They treat almost all the referred patients as addicts. The problem with this is less than a third of them might have a remote chance of actually being one.

The problem, then, for treatment centers is that if they are treating addicts, they must tell them they have "a disease." However, if the patient is not actually an addict but did occasionally or even repeatedly binge-drink or abuse drugs, how is he or she going to respond to traditional disease/addiction treatment?

According to most research, it seems, not very well.

The majority of people I saw in meetings, referred there by a treatment center, were situational abusers. Make no mistake; it is a condition that can be serious, even deadly. Nonetheless, it helps no one if the abuser is left to fend for him- or herself alone, as is too often the case if he or she doesn't fall into the AA model. Instead, we'll have another treatment-failure back out on the street, using again.

Who is "getting helped" then? Surprisingly, many of these "patients" found relief for their drinking/drug problem on their own. It is a concept called "moderation," also known as self-control or common sense! Some drinkers/drug abusers, however, will respond well to the "blanket approach" of today's recovery—and after several relapses on their own—will come back to AA, join up, and stay on.

I did.

There is much benefit to this: belonging to a club that is actually happy to have you as a member. I was, in the late comic Groucho Marx's category of club-joiners: he often said he "would not belong to any organization that would have allowed him to be a member!"

There was this, too: I'd alienated most of my friends and family network through repeated bad behavior and other errors in judgment. AA was my club of last resort. It was pretty cool to be welcomed back to AA over and over until I gradually accepted the idea: this might work for me too.

I had joined AA the last time after having been treated as an inpatient at a major treatment center for excessive marijuana use. A pothead now allowed in "Alcoholics Anonymous"? We're talking about a new AA. All addictions and abuses are welcome. You just simply become "chemically dependent," and no one will ever question you about belonging there. A lot of people who need help but are not necessarily alcoholic make their way to AA.

Let's then look at how I did it.

Chapter 4
A Troubled Youth

The road of life that led me to AA had many bumps and turns. Each of us is the germination of a life-collection of experiences and knowledge gained, as expressed so well in the words of the band the Grateful Dead: "What a long strange trip it's been."

1957. I went through my adolescence in the late '50s and early '60s. The boys I'd grown up with all became either greasers or baldies. I favored the early Elvis look—definitely greaser. With a tall leanness, at almost six feet and 165 lbs, I pulled it off along with the boys I ran with, in a place called "the Bluff."

It overlooked the Burlington Northern railroad yards with many adjacent mills and factories. The homes there were small- to medium-sized, prewar, working-class dwellings. Looking back, it seems to me there was a windblown look about them, faded paint, weathered siding. Most of the streets were shaded by huge, spreading elm trees, giving either a continual somberness, or, when the sun's shafts pierced the leafy canopy, a cathedral majesty to the streets and alleyways there.

Summer evenings were often tinged with fine soot. If the breeze was from the southwest, as it often was, a pungent, diesel-locomotive burning smell mixed with creosote also hung in the air, which made for an airborne, toxic cocktail. I loved that place.

For kids, summers on the Bluff were spent climbing the cliffs over the railroad tracks and enjoying the freedom of riding our bicycles everywhere we pleased. We were out of our houses in the early morning and didn't return until dinnertime. However, some of us were truly not safe at all.

A sixteen-year-old neighbor who lived three doors up the street, Bobby, had recently obtained a driver's license. I was only twelve years old and was fascinated with the new pale-green Buick Roadmaster automobile his father had recently acquired. Bobby had full use of it, I learned. A powerful V8 motor imparted deep, resonant vibrations as it growled at idle. "Would you like a ride?" he asked.

"Yes," I answered. He asked for just one small favor in return. It involved sex, but he cajoled, "We'll just do some fooling around." That he was four years older than twelve-year-old me made it an "abuse of a minor" case, if it ever came to that. It should have, but it never did.

Out Highway 12 a few miles, there was an abandoned shack on the property that his parents had purchased to build a new home on. We could go out there to smoke some cigarettes, which I liked, and "have some fun." Riding in his (not Mom's or Dad's) car and smoking cigarettes was all I heard. The trap was set. Off we went, but what I didn't know was that he was a predator.

Afterward, I hated him and myself for a long time. My parents did find out I had gone for a ride with him and forbade me from seeing him again. They never found out about his taking advantage of me; to my best recall, they never asked. No, check that; they did ask:

"What did you do?"

"We were just riding around?"

"You were gone so long. What were you thinking, going off like that?"

I couldn't answer; I was so ashamed and humiliated.

Bobby added insult to injury as he stalked me and harassed me off and on for years! I got wise to him, though, and learned to duck him after I saw what he was about. Years later, it seems Bobby finally cured himself of his problem. He died in what the local newspaper reported as an accidental poisoning at his job in a chemical company. I will always wonder if it was self-inflicted.

A year after my ride with Bobby, several things happened in quick succession to diffuse and blur the situation in my ADD-addled mind.

First, my mom delivered the baby girl we three older brothers had been waiting for; this is a happy memory, caring for my little sister, a lot! Feeding, changing, and rocking her to sleep. We are still close.

Shortly after this, my parents announced we were moving, away from the only home I'd ever known, to a rambler out in the suburbs.

Then, within weeks of those two events, my grandmother, who had lived with us and doted on me since my birth, died suddenly at age sixty-six. It was she who I'd formed my maternal bond with because my mother had unfortunately been ill for the first year of my life. To be clear here, I did love my mother, but the maternal bond I had with my grandma never really formed between Mom and me.

Now, just having turned thirteen, I was starting over with a new neighborhood, new friends, and new school, and with my maternal grandmother gone from my life. I was reeling, as out of control as I had ever felt. Thank God for my two younger brothers and new baby sister, I did not live in a vacuum. However I know my ADD behavior affected them.

Earlier in my life—in first grade, I believe—I was thought to have an advanced intellect because of my erratic behavior. Decades later, I would learn of my condition, now known as ADD (attention deficit disorder). At the time, however, this behavior in a small boy was seen as evidence of being undisciplined, having a short attention span, and, you know, being otherwise, smart!

The result was that they, unbelievably, moved me ahead one full grade—from first to third. This move was coupled with my transfer from a beautiful granite building standing in and named after Mounds Park (public school), a still favored place, to a Catholic school. This did not make life any easier for me or anyone near me. Instead of getting the satisfaction of completing schoolwork well, I was now usually behind and getting the "what's wrong with you" lecture.

I struggled with all of the usual adolescent plights, especially puberty. (*Catholics then were against exercising it.*)

My mother never forgot that one of the nuns remarked to her at a parent-teacher event, "I just don't know what gets into him sometimes."

Eighth grade concluded with the aforementioned events of Bobby the pervert encroaching into, and Grandmother departing from, my life, etc. More drama would follow through ninth grade at another new school.

A teacher named Brother Theodore, my ninth grade Spanish teacher at the just-opened Mary T. Hill Catholic High School, long since merged into Hill Murray High School, helped me to center "my focus" one day early in the new school year when he asked why I hadn't turned in my homework. My reply must have offended him. Bam, bam! I was caught off guard by the left, then right, open-handed slaps delivered to my soft, youthful face, which at the time was covering a mouth full of new metal braces! The shock and pain were horrible, not to mention the embarrassment.

I was sent to the office, where I was immediately transferred out of Spanish into study hall. I never saw Brother Theodore again. I avoided contact with him until the end of the school year, when I informed my parents that if I weren't allowed to transfer (back) to the local public high school, they likely would never see me again. No frivolous threat here—I was adamant.

I had run away earlier in late summer just after we had moved into the new house, for a night and a day, acting out on a rage I didn't know how to tell anyone about. My poor parents were terrified, as I know now.

In spite of or because of my hysterics, they complied, and I began tenth grade much more contentedly than I had begun ninth. It has been, remarkably, fifty years since those days, and I must confess, if I ran into Brother Theodore again, he'd still have some serious answering to do for me. I am continually amazed at the human capacity to retain resentment even of a slight that hasn't been visited for these long decades.

(Ah then, I feel a bit better now. Allow me to return the reader to my ADD-influenced life.)

Except for a change in the way discipline was administered (thank goodness), high school was otherwise not much different. A lackluster event day after day, except for my continuous acting-out, causing disruptions and fights and antagonizing teachers who didn't see me as just bored and trying to be funny. The assistant principal and I became pals at his time-out sessions for me. Years later, I sold him a life insurance policy, and we shared a few chuckles.

1963. Before my senior year was completed, I dropped out and enlisted in the navy. In the middle of my basic training, November, President Kennedy was killed. This led to a conscious awakening to my youthful, naïve mind. I recall feeling remarkably vulnerable but comforted somewhat by my circumstances as a serviceman. This too, was to be short-lived.

A couple months later, I reported to the San Diego navy base to board a ship (which had already departed). I wasn't late; it left early.

The TV in the lounge was blasting the Beatles on their first *Ed Sullivan Show* appearance. For the next several months, I would hear them, the Rolling Stones, Elvis, and Frankie Valley, as I was drinking beers in saloons all over the parts of Asia I visited. This drinking occurred during the search for my assigned ship, when I briefly toured the Far East. There, eighteen-year-old US servicemen were allowed to spend money in saloons that would be off-limits at home, imbibing adult beverages while on leave in local villages and towns. Local, professional bawdy girls were likewise available. I had been thrust into a "Hollywood movie" of a freewheeling adventurer's life. I took advantage of these opportunities as often as possible.

What was surreal, even then, was that I would not have a drinking privilege when I returned to the states, as I was too young, while scores of my peers were being sent to Vietnam, regardless of their youth. I never got recalled for that assignment.

Sadly, within a year, after repeated visits to sick bay, I was released from active duty and granted an honorable discharge. The cause was chronic bronchitis, which was reoccurring so often they had to let me out. This condition eventually cleared up on its own. I never found out why it happened in the first place. The tropics are a cause for some.

Too bad more of my American comrades didn't suffer the same fate instead of conscription to serve in Vietnam, which I would now avoid.

Because of the escalating war in Vietnam, the navy was putting warships into service at a rapid rate. They were not hand-selecting crews; the wholesale stocking of ships was more necessary. Luckily for me, my illness had made me unfit for sea duty.

Another unexpected new beginning. Arriving back home, still only eighteen, meant no more unhindered drinking for me, not for at least three more years. Taking all of this as a new challenge, I started getting my life in order. I earned a high school diploma at night school, learned a trade as a drafter, and got a job in a large architectural office.

The Vietnam War was expanding, as were the protests against it. I wanted to support the war effort. I had had many high school friends who were drafted into the service to fight over there. Many of them did not come back, and many who did had lost their youth and some, their ability to reason rationally through drug addiction. Therefore, protesting the conflict while remaining a patriot became a constant struggle.

One of my friends, a boyhood pal named Roger, was always the kind of guy who could not settle for second best and had always wanted to be a marine. Innocence lost is all I can think of when recalling how he was before he left and then after he returned. But how, I wonder, could it have been otherwise?

Never mind what I thought; Roger was in his element. He could have been a poster model for Marine Corps recruiting; he loved it, and it showed. Vietnam was waiting, and he was ready to go to serve "over there." From high school on, he had always been a quiet, serious guy blessed with a good sense of humor. When he returned from Vietnam, those traits were gone, and he had become cynical, morose, and jumpy.

He told us a few hair-raising stories of things he had witnessed in Vietnam. Those memories had taken the fun out of his life. He often told us he could no longer enjoy things as he used to since seeing the real face of evil in the war.

Somehow, he finally met a beautiful, raven-haired girl named Sharon. Shortly after, they unexpectedly had a "quickie" wedding. After disappearing from our lives for several months, he returned one day to sadly announce she had left him. We never found out why. She just went away.

Roger then reenlisted in the marines and went back to Vietnam for another tour. Two years later, when he returned for the last time, he was even more a shadow of the man he had been. He took second- and third-shift jobs to seclude himself even further, I believe. I would try to get together with him, meet with some of our friends, but it was clear he had no heart for it.

At the end, the last couple of years, he was out of touch with me. One day I heard he had died some months ago. In my heart, I knew he had really left us a long time ago in a foreign place far, far away, like a lot of other Rogers before him had.

Until now, I have never paid Roger the homage he deserved. *I tip my hat to you, old friend. I will always cherish the memory I have of you.*

More amends are needed here to my brothers and sister: Please know this—I take full responsibility for alienating you during these early adult years of my life. ADD frequently travels without a conscience, and I was usually looking out for my own best interests (pleasures). In the process, I left my family behind.

I watched you all grow up and grow into your lives, all of you talented. Ken, so smart with things mechanical, quiet, thoughtful, strong, like our father. John, intuitive and quick-minded, funny and gifted with an ability to commune with animals and people. Nancy, caring, thoughtful, strong, and terribly loyal to all those near her, especially our parents in their declining years. She has become a close friend.

I struggled in the late '60s with the war, drug culture, "anything goes" lifestyle, more loose women than I had ever seen before. There were too many distractions and no real focus for my life other than getting as much of what I thought was my share as I could. I left a lot of responsibilities behind.

Chapter 5
Adulthood, More Trouble

1969. I was now nineteen. Irresponsible behavior reared its ugly head more and more in my life. I had been "hanging out" with another boyhood pal, Greg, doing a lot of binge drinking and now smoking pot, when we could get it. His girlfriend joined us.

Sheila was a high-spirited girl, and it would be a lie to say this wasn't fun. Sometimes I would even bring along other girls I had met to share the party with us. Sheila, very tolerant, even seemed to enjoy these experiences. *Seemed* is the key word here.

Actions oftentimes do have consequences, and this partying cost her and Greg their marriage, and their little son lost his daddy. One day Sheila left, took the boy ran away, literally and disappeared. No one ever saw them again. Greg claims he tried but could not find them. I do not believe him.

Reviewing this history of mine through the dim mists of years gone by and memories faded, I still believe I was not an alcoholic, as I would later declare myself, although I did drink and use marijuana frequently, abuse is not always addiction, and neither is low tolerance for alcoholic beverages. Much more likely for me, it was the continuance of this ADD personality quirk, which had been showing itself since my youth.

Thanks to my low tolerance for alcohol, coupled with a lack of self-discipline, I had had my share of drinking events since returning from the navy years earlier. I had even managed to get myself arrested and jailed, twice in the same hot summer. But I don't know if these incidences were ever as much drunken episodes as they were youthful stupidity.

The first episode was excessive speed; the cop clocked me at over one hundred miles an hour in a thirty-five-mile an hour zone, after 1:30 a.m. He locked me in his police cruiser's backseat almost as fast. My car was towed to impound. I was released the following morning with a future court date for a speeding ticket but not for drunk driving!

A couple of months later, another event—drag racing on a downtown street and then, this time, smart-mouthing the arresting officer. Ironically, neither time was I arrested for being drunk. Just for behaving stupidly and for speeding. This time, however, I did lose my license for a year, and my new car was now gone forever. No license and no need for it either.

1970. Now twenty-four, with my driving privileges intact, I was still working in an architect's office. I met the woman who would become my first wife while out barhopping, and soon after this, I asked her to marry and she accepted. Six months later we were wed, which leads to more drinking stories including the following: I got drunk at the groom's dinner, I got fairly drunk at the wedding, and I may have drunk too much on our honeymoon.

About a year after we married, she demanded we attend marriage counseling. This may have had something to do with my drinking, too, but not exclusively. There was a surprise coming. It also happened that we had gotten pregnant. We were both overjoyed. I did drink a highball or two most evenings. Again, it was never about getting knocked-out, just getting a buzz on.

Why get a buzz on? Good question.

My father had had a beer or two most evenings after work, often one before dinner. He'd still go to work every day too. I never recall seeing Dad drunk, not even once in the more than sixty years I was privileged to know him.

I had briefly drunk with guys who wanted to drink to oblivion, and occasionally I ended up being their driver. This kind of binge drinking never made sense to me—especially after I tried it and found the hangovers were horrible. Truth be told, it had frequently seemed like a good idea to have only a drink or two, not more. What was often missing for me, however, were the personal limitations, also known as self-control.

Note: To better make the case for my claim of irresponsible drinking behavior, not "addiction," I ask myself this: Could I ever have had as good a time on less or even on no beverage alcohol at all?

Certainly, and often I did.

But in all honesty, usually I simply didn't try to. Back then, I wasn't exercising much caution and often did have one too many. Here, too, I did spend many pleasant moments: working on my latest hot rod car, which I loved to polish, detail, and fuss with; taking long bicycle rides; reading; playing sports such as Frisbee, swimming, sailing, or hiking; or enjoying my diverse music collection of jazz, classics, and pop. I loved everything from Sinatra to Bach and Ray Charles to the Rolling Stones.

I had also attended further night school for architectural education for years. I did have a life other than getting high. Frequently, I would fall asleep in front of the TV or while reading or listening to my record collection on the component stereo system I had acquired piece by piece.

This regularly happened while being somewhat isolated under my prized Koss headphones. My wife often just put the baby to bed and then went to bed without me. Even so, frequently waking up those mornings, alone in the living room, is not the way I'd imagined married life to be, but again, why not—what's the harm? It seemed to irritate her, though. I guess it didn't fit her idea of married life either.

Note: For most of the past forty-plus years, I have still frequently fallen asleep alone in front of the TV (my new wife had gone to bed too). This happened even through the years I attended AA, during which I did not drink anything.

Chapter 6
Beverly Hills' AA in Minnesota

1975. I'd lost my drafting job due to the economy. The '70s were tough this way. A lot of us were out of work, and selling cars was the best option I could find at the time. I went to work every day, regardless of how hungover. Ah, youth. Not excusing anything; just reporting what happened.

I would attend my first AA meeting in the autumn, and it was such a sweet seduction. I'd been married a couple of years by now, had my one son, and had become fairly successful at selling cars in a down economy, thanks, also, to some high-pressure sales managers in the car dealership. This, after more than ten years slaving as a drafter in the large architectural office, seemed much more satisfying too.

While liking the people contact, I loathed sales failures. Personal rejection is a curse that still pursues me.

Also at the dealership was another used-car jockey named Steve who befriended me. He also had noticed my frequently hungover condition, especially at the Saturday morning sales meetings. Being a hyper type of controlling person and a long-time member of AA, he zeroed in on hapless me. He somehow convinced me that quitting was the only way to end the hangovers and drug withdrawals and that going to AA meetings was the only way to quit.

Wanting his approval more than anything, I accepted his invitation to go along to his regular Friday night AA meeting. I found Steve to be a gregarious fellow and had laughed a lot with him. We both liked to flirt with the ladies too. Yes, he also was married. Truth be told, I wasn't thinking seriously about quitting drinking, I mostly went along to hang out with the otherwise-often-reticent Steve!

It was a very prestigious AA group located in one of the tonier suburbs. This Lake Minnetonka neighborhood was a version of Beverly Hills, close enough to the real thing even in Minnesota. It has rolling hills, gated communities, mansions on the lakeshore, and yachts.

The parking lot was filled with mostly high-end, late-model vehicles, especially Cadillacs, Mercedes-Benzes, Corvettes, Porsches, and even a Maserati or two. Was I impressed? Yes, and it was just the beginning.

Soon, when I was seated in my very first AA meeting with these apparently really rich people, it was confirmed in my mind. These folks seemed to be just what *I wanted to be like*.

As a poor boy from the lower East Side, I had known of many wealthy people. As a youth, I was a caddie at a nearby private golf club for three summers. Lots of moneyed golfers belonged there. I grew to like wealthy people; they were generally laid-back, and they tipped well. Also, as a recovering Catholic, I learned how to take this envy of others' wealth very seriously.

Inside the Lake Minnetonka Saint-Something Church basement, the AA meeting was just getting started. I had no idea of what to expect; Steve hadn't told me much. Steve only ever told anyone just what he needed him or her to hear anyway. Typical for a used-car sales veteran.

The AA meeting wasn't unlike an informal church service, as it opened with the serenity prayer, which set a nice sentiment. The meeting began with us all together in one large church dining room, where I was brought into the proceedings and introduced as a "new member," and everyone said:

"Hi, Howard."

The group then organized a "newcomers'" meeting, and a dozen of them were separated off into a smaller room with me. Steve didn't join us, which I found a little disloyal. Since he had coerced me into coming, he should at least stay for the execution, I thought. Going around the table, most of the people told a short version of their drunk-a-logs; some just gave their first name, stated they were an alcoholic, and then passed.

Some of the ones who spoke had fascinating stories to tell. Many had achieved success in life, which preached to what I had always been looking for. One particular member, Terry, told of a summer dinner party he had held at his home on the shore of Lake Minnetonka, with famous visiting rock band members.

We were all shocked to find out who they were. At this party, Terry had become so inebriated he was seriously in danger of injuring someone. He had driven his golf cart, drunk, through the crowd, and, finally, into the lake! Someone had called the cops. I thought, *Even Lake Minnetonka drunks can get arrested* and was mildly surprised at this.

I tried really hard to empathize with Terry. I had seen Lake Minnetonka up close a few times and had always found it very impressive. I also liked the idea of a guest rock band; who wouldn't? Further, since I too had been arrested a couple of times, all in all, this entire AA thing looked promising.

Others at the table told of how they discovered they couldn't drink alcohol with impunity either. So after getting in trouble from overimbibing, they eventually went on to admit that they too were "powerless over alcohol" and then got on with the AA program. And, it seemed good fortune had followed after many of them here; good jobs, prestige, hooking up with noteworthy people. And there you have it—"success, success, success!"

All of this they had achieved once they sobered up and crawled out of the pathetic gutter, jail, detox center, hospital bed, psychiatric ward, or treatment center they had found themselves in.

Their recovery had also stopped them from having suicidal thoughts or actual attempts, some claimed, or it had just eased the general feeling of low self-esteem! This was all good too. All of these wonderful things and more had started happening to them, I'd heard, over and over, when they had begun following the teachings of Alcoholics Anonymous. Seriously, this is what almost all of them said had happened. They'd gathered together—"one day at a time"—toward becoming the successful, sober people you saw them as today.

Hallelujah!

I was as envious as I had ever been in my life! I was positively green with envy, of these drunks, as they called themselves. Also, at the beginning of the meeting, I'd heard a convincing passage read from Chapter 5, "How It Works," in the Big Book of Alcoholics Anonymous: "If you have decided that you want what we have and are willing to go to any lengths to get it…"

Any lengths? I was sick and tired of being broke and feeling like a loser and was ready *to try literally anything* to get what they had, even if the anything part meant giving up using drugs and alcohol!

Note: Not so coincidentally, I learned that *this is the **only** way **anyone** does get and stay sober, in or out of Alcoholics Anonymous. If you want it (recovery) bad enough, you **can** do it!* First, you have to decide for yourself that you want to quit drinking or using. In other words, *AA* *doesn't make you quit.* Let me repeat this salient point: Alcoholics Anonymous does not *mystically* make you stop drinking!

The point again is only you can make this decision and only when you are ready to—and not one minute sooner! As I said earlier, AA simply gives you a place to meet with "like-minded" people who need to quit drinking and using too.

There really is nothing magical about this. Do not misunderstand what was just said here; what I had discovered through Steve and the Lake Minnetonka AA meeting was pretty much what I would find—at every AA meeting—for the next thirty-five years. This is not to say something good isn't happening here. But, it turns out, what is actually happening, in my opinion, is not what AA tells you it is. I happened to decide to begin to abstain, while there, *on my own,* not because of anything AA said or did.

What if a member insists (as many do) that a "spiritual experience" caused him or her to quit? Then has it not become a religion with a capital *R*?

But AA always claims it is not a religion.

However, if you were to ask one of the AA "old-timers" about this, he or she would, in all likelihood, tell you to "just keep coming back." This is fine, too, as long as it makes sense to you. Sometimes people just need to quit abusing drugs and alcohol no matter how they achieve this.

Years later, I attended an annual statewide AA convention. Thousands of members were there. Each group had a hospitality suite; I wandered into the Lake Minnetonka AA club's room and saw a few people I'd met at my first meeting. When I inquired about Steve, Terry, and some others, I found they had not been seen in years.

Chapter 7
What I Found AA to Be Like, at First

1975. The following week, I attended another in a long line of local, church-basement AA meetings near my home on the west side of the city. I would continue to go to meetings there until a year or so later, when I moved to the Summit Avenue AA meeting, held in a beautiful mansion on the famous street in St. Paul where local author F. Scott Fitzgerald had lived. I would attend the Wednesday evening meeting there for the next three years.

Other improvements in my life continued. The hangovers ceased immediately, never to return. I made some new friends, a lot of local people, who were very nice but not nearly as affluent as the Lake Minnetonka AA crowd. The envy thing again? I didn't stop searching for an answer.

As time went by, I began to notice the AA community did have its share of the semi notorious: thieves, con artists, hustlers, drug dealers, and even occasional celebrities. It was the nature of the beast in those days, especially with so many of these characters all in one place. It seemed to me that a lot of people wanted to be seen getting sober. For a while then, it was the thing to do. Even Elvis and Clapton were rumored to have been treated at Hazel-butt, as we referred to the treatment center up the road in Center City.

I did meet many local celebrities in AA, including a former University of Minnesota football star who had shared a famous Gopher football team with a later, former NFL head coach and a famous professional wrestler. Later on, I got to know other famous and notable people: TV and radio personalities who were taking a break from their overindulgent behavior, much as I was, and had joined this club of nondrinkers called AA.

Thirty plus years later, some of these guys can still impress with their stature. I had never before run across such a privileged microcosm of society. Did the treatment centers have influence on their being here? No doubt. Again, a few short years later, there were none to be seen any longer or even heard about. The fad had passed.

Each week, my group would meet in this large former private residence. We were a dozen or so men and often one or two women. We were dissimilar to the meeting I have described at the Lake Minnetonka AA in the previous chapter. We held a small group meeting and kept the opening brief. Many other AA clubs operate this way, too.

Occasionally we had a sobriety-recognition ceremony, and a medallion award was given to one of the group's members. These were meaningful events for me and continued to be so for many years. It was moving to see someone whose life had been in chaos quit using drugs or alcohol, then continue to attend weekly meetings and follow-the-steps, as it's called, and subsequently repair his or her life.

For those who eventually achieve this state in life—almost nobody does it at first or even after several attempts—it is a meaningful achievement.

Upstairs, in what had certainly been a bedroom—now ringed with chairs and tables, all well-kept—the setting was very unlike the old downtown AA club meetings. We each brought in a coffee and found a place to perch. The meeting here always began with the serenity prayer. Then the designated squad leader began by reading the step we would discuss this evening. We went through one each of the twelve steps weekly.

Each one in turn, commented on the step's impact on his or her life, and then passed to the next person to share his or her thoughts or experiences with the practice of it also. Each individual spoke for three to five minutes.

We tried to complete the discussions in just over an hour. Many who spoke had *not* actually achieved the task given in the step but regaled us with how they would go about it—*someday*. We suffered through those, too.

Other differences with the downtown AA meeting, which was an audience attended format only: everybody spoke here, and noticeably more and more of us claimed to be *chemically dependent* in contrast to those identified as *alcoholics*.

If, for some reason, we lacked the ability to speak on the subject at hand, we passed after giving our name and disease statement. Most did not pass, as they had something they felt needed to be said. Some were amusing; a couple were painfully boring (those people tended to drone on and on). I've seen some go longer than twenty minutes!

In an AA meeting, rarely does anyone ask, "Why are we doing this?" The simple answer would be, "Because it is what has always been done—talking about our problems through the propriety of the Steps." Other non-step groups with dissimilar motives such as "feelings meetings" might call them *talking points*. The Steps keep everyone on-topic—the recovery of drug or alcohol abuse.

Here I have grouped my fellow meeting members into three categories:

First. The true believers, who believe they know why they are there, make up about a third.

Second. Those who are trying to assimilate, to fit in to see if this will work (this time), make up a few more of us.

Third. Those who "don't give-a-shit" at all about any of this recovery crap and are not at all happy to be court-ordered there are relatively rare, often only one or two of the members.

Over the next thirty years, this balance did not shift perceptibly. The meetings did work for me too, for a long time. Then one day, it just didn't matter enough anymore.

Chapter 8
When AA Changed Forever

1960. An investigative newspaper story of **AA** might have (quite accurately) reported thusly:

"If your addiction is drugs, not alcohol, do not waste your time going to Alcoholics Anonymous!"

It seems drug addicts, marijuana smokers, heroin addicts, pill poppers and all other chemically dependent people need not have applied for help here.

Why not, you may ask?

Because early on, AA was a private society. It had a clear restriction on who could and could not attend its meetings. Closed meetings, meaning "alcoholics only" were the standard for more than thirty years after the group was formed as "Alcoholics Anonymous" in 1935. Prior to then, it had been known as "The Oxford Groupers," an arguably for-profit, Protestant, Christian abstinence society also known as; "Buchman's Millionaires" because of the penchant of their leader, the Rev. Frank Buchman, for recruiting wealthy patrons into his private, but well-funded society.

1970. The new decade brought soldiers returning from Vietnam, and, of course, the new counterculture drug addicts and casual drug abusers who accumulated with them. This group became more frequently noticed at AA meetings. There, they were often told, "Drug addicts should seek out a NA (Narcotics Anonymous) meeting; we at AA are here for alcoholics only. We are a closed meeting." If any druggies were bold enough to linger, they were often treated less than welcomingly. I know this firsthand because it happened in my own AA meetings.

The "chemically dependent" members who dominate AA meetings today, **were not welcome at AA** for its first several decades of existence! We argued endlessly about this with our local AA club's steering committees in the mid-1970s. Each week, dozens more of the drug-abuse or "chemically dependent" referrals showed up as first-timers to AA. We could not keep turning them away. What changed, you may ask? Well, the enormous influence of the $5-billion-a-year treatment center industry is what.

When the treatment centers sprang up like used car lots in the 1970s, they needed credibility, and AA gave it to them instantly. It was, however, a lot like going to a Mack truck dealer for your next new vehicle. Mack may make a stout dump truck, but its minivan and sports car programs are severely lacking.

This was the quandary that had overwhelmed the AA of "for alcoholics only" fame: overnight, AA was being touted as this one-size-fits-all solution. This large net, I believe, contributes to the previously mentioned "revolving door" you still see in AA meetings everywhere. The dirty little secret nobody talks about is this: using AA in this catchall capacity isn't working very well, and the statistics show it.

1992. A *Wikipedia* article titled "Effectiveness of Alcoholics Anonymous" reported the results of several studies, including the 1990 National Longitudinal Alcohol Epidemiologic Survey[1] (NLAES). Of the 43,000 surveys sent out to the AA clubs, more than 1,100 of AA attendees responded.

The NLAES discovered that only **31 percent of members continued attending AA meetings with regularity**. Later, AA's triennial surveys backed up this number in more depth. There were other surveys: PEALE, CASPAR, NIAAA, etc.

All of these surveys conclude, more or less, that about a third of AA members remain sober for **"some number of years."** The treatment centers and AA alike now welcome everyone: druggies and drunks alike, nonconformists, dropouts, and social rejects—anyone really.

Today, more than three decades after I first joined, I personally find AA to be at least one of three things:

1. It can be one of the better places to recover, *if you truly have the symptoms* of the disease of alcoholism.
2. However, more than 90 percent of new referrals to AA are in a continual exodus, running for the doors, perhaps because they have discovered AA's claims of recovery are overstated. (Or could it be that both statements might be correct?)
3. Or, *AA might no longer be necessary as it exists today!*

To the first point: what AA has been good at for some, as little as 10 percent, (surveys vary between 10 & 30%) of its members is to provide a meeting place for those who have decided they need to quit *excessively* drinking or taking drugs, enabling them to gather together and share this experience with other like-minded people.

Again, "If you love AA and feel it's working for you, you do not need to read this book any further!

To address the second point based on the research I spoke of: what AA is equally bad at is trying to require everyone who partakes of it to accept the concept that they have a disease they are supposedly powerless over!

Some do, to be sure, but everyone? Not according to the files of police, courts, parole officers, county hospitals, and treatment centers. They all keep records of arrests, bookings, sentencing, admitting, referrals, insurance evaluations, etc. When these files are examined for "alcohol-related incidents," a public record of recidivism is found. And as far as AA's recovery record is concerned, it is not great. Studies of these public records have mirrored the CASPAR one I spoke of earlier. Recovery does occur for approximately 31 percent of AA members "someday, eventually," but not at the beginning; at the outset, recovery is actually less than 3 percent.

The ones who finally do come back to stay in AA only do so after much "trial and failure." To their credit, the many who have made this long walk have enriched their own lives and the lives of fellow AA regulars. They are part of the 31 percent of members in attendance at AA meetings on any given day.

What about the third point? About AA being unnecessary?

There is a universal formula used for determining whether someone has an alcohol/drug addiction, which is this:

Repetition of a behavior equals a pattern of abuse.

This is what supposedly separates the alcoholics from the so-called abusers. For instance, most of the rest of us, alcohol and drug users (or abusers), are of the "average temperate drinker" variety referred to by Dr. William D. Silkworth in his "description of an alcoholic" in the original 1939 text of the book *Alcoholics Anonymous.* Does simply overindulging or binge drinking too often make us addicts or just abusers in the eyes of the recovery industry? In a word, addicts.

Often, AA clubs, as they are called, are a haven for both addicts and abusers to gather side by side with regular citizens, working-class folks, housewives, corporate climbers, unemployed, students, welfare recipients, and street people, etc. All now make up this most diverse organization.

So, what's the harm? Well, the huge dropout numbers, for one thing; you know, the fact that two-thirds of the newcomers run for the door, never to return.

Why?

I believe by the time they get to treatment and are referred to AA, they learn about AA's originally stated goal, which is *"helping alcoholics to achieve sobriety."*

Today, this seems very noble, but allowing virtually anyone to join would have AA's founders rolling over in their graves. Their baby—this AA thing—was NOT created to help *other-than-alcoholic* members, period!

Nowhere in the preface or within the first five chapters of the original text of the Big Book of Alcoholics Anonymous, originally published in 1939, is "drug addiction" or "chemical dependency" mentioned at all.

AA was created to remedy alcoholism! Drug use was an aside, if mentioned at all. Which is why it seems to be such a bad fit for so many of the new referrals from courts, parole officers, treatment centers, etc.—but fit it must—because as far as the recovery industry is concerned, it's practically the only game in town!

It used to be that chemically dependent people did not fit into AA's criteria of an alcoholic. Many of them are cured of their heroin addiction but still seem to drink socially. Many of the Narc-Anon attendees would meet at a local saloon for beers after their NA meeting concluded.

We used to tell the *chemically dependent* referrals they needed to go elsewhere. The other reasons for the differences are many. We'll cover the main one next, the AA description of the cure itself.

When it comes to the use of alcohol or recreational drugs, personal responsibility and moderation are never on the table for AA members.

Why not?

Because, I believe, with the application of self-control, mind control is no longer relevant! For instance, through its twelve-step program, AA attempts to help its members rein in every other area of their lives—relationships, sex urges, self-control, etc. And yet AA also says ***moderate use is something we are not able to control***.[2] AA can say it, but most of the newcomers are not buying it, and the recidivism statistics don't support it either.

AA was created to treat alcoholics and if they are not the same as the chemically dependent or casual abusers, who are they then? Let's look at what they call their fix.

Chapter 9
The AA Cure

2014. What seems to scare most of these newcomers away from AA meetings is hearing the intentions of *Alcoholics Anonymous*, with this reading given at the opening of most AA meetings everywhere: "Rarely have we seen a person fail, who has thoroughly followed our path…"[1]

Why would AA make a statement like this at the opening of each meeting? Answer (again) in three parts.

Part One. Because the "our path" AA is referring to will supposedly lead to the cure! This is found in the AA twelve steps at number 3, where we "Made a decision to turn our will and our lives over to the care of God as we understand him."[2]

Simply stated, the *"cure"* for alcoholism is *asking God to "take over" and fix it*.

The entire program just wouldn't make any sense otherwise. Why? See part two for my explanation.)

Part Two. AA requires you to admit *your abuse is caused by a disease that causes insanity*!

Really?

Yes, that is exactly what they are saying: that you have abused drink (drugs not mentioned) because you are insane! This, too, is clearly stated in AA's twelve steps at number two, where we must eventually "Come to believe that a power greater than ourselves could restore us to sanity."

Part Three. Furthermore, when you, as an AA member agreed to the first proposition, you claimed this ***needs to be so***, as AA states in step number one: "We admitted that we were powerless over alcohol; that our lives had become unmanageable."

That's why!

Just in case you missed it, the point here is in step number one, rephrased: *"We admitted to having no control over our drinking alcohol!"*

How about, why NOT say: "I am not going to be an alcoholic drinker? Or, more simply, say; "I am not going to drink excessively." Instead, what AA has us saying is this: "I cannot drink alcohol because I am powerless to manage my intake of it, because when it comes to drinking it, I must be insane!"

For the Lefty Bs (chapter 1) and other hard-core drinkers of the world, this probably makes sense, but casual abusers or stupid or youthful binge-drinkers are initially or eventually repelled by this reasoning, and then they do not listen to the message any longer.

So, for a solution, why not say: "I won't use alcohol and/or drugs any longer because it causes me problems" (and so I am going to become a nonuser)?

It is a much more positive statement, which also states that we are in control of our own lives.

The majority of us, in fact, *do* do this.

Again, while AA's original concept sounds like a noble goal, almost nobody ever actually does give up drinking alcohol at first, not without backsliding a whole bunch of times. And this matters a lot to a newcomer who is desperately looking for help.

AA's cofounder Bill Wilson actually admitted this publicly at the funeral of Dr. Bob Smith, his partner and cofounder of AA, after nearly seventeen years of the existence of the fellowship. He stated while giving the eulogy, "We went through over 100 prospects before finding even one who was willing to follow this plan."

However, they *never* changed a word of their initial plan.

Why AA Is Not a Universal Recovery Treatment

Let's continue with an analysis of the "Introduction to AA" reading, as this is where the heavy logic is brought out to influence a decision. Here is an excerpt from the opening of Chapter 5, which states, *"Rarely have we seen a person fail, who has thoroughly followed our path,* those who do not recover are people who cannot or will not completely give themselves to this simple program, usually men and women who are **constitutionally incapable of being honest with themselves**"!

Say what, please?

Well, they are saying in a not-so-subtle way that if you do not swallow whole this AA twelve-step concept and then recover (quit using), the **fault is in your own lack of character**, not in what they offer as a "cure."

This is "the why" of my argument about AA not being the universal recovery treatment for many people, especially those, who as far as we know, had exercised some bad judgment about their situational drug and/or alcohol use, got into trouble, and came to AA for help—voluntarily or otherwise.

I recall the dozens of court-ordered DUI (driving under the influence) referrals I sponsored. They all admitted to being stupid about drinking and driving, and they faithfully attended AA as their court-ordered sentence requirement. Almost none continued on in AA when it ended, however.

We occasionally saw some of them return because of a second DUI, but it was more likely they were jailed long-term after the next drunk driving arrest. You see, jail will keep you sober, too, even without treatment or AA meetings. Imagine today, if a doctor treating you for any ailment (other than drug addiction) gave you the same explanation AA uses, which, simply stated, is "just take our word for it," while pronouncing that you will likely not survive your illness after all! As Sgt. Joe Friday on TV's *Dragnet* used to say, "Just the facts ma'am, just the facts."

Well, the fact here is you drank too much. How about not doing this anymore? No more excuses like "I can't, it's not my fault, and I'm powerless." How about this instead: don't binge-drink, guzzle your drinks, and, especially, don't (then) drive a vehicle.

What I learned after quitting AA, is moderation management of my alcohol intake. It works like this:

Police yourself with the first drink; check the time and make sure you will not have a second one for at least an hour or more. Then, if you make sure you eat some food, you likely won't get intoxicated. A third one much later, occasionally is possible. But if you think you are tipsy, don't drive your car!

You don't need treatment for some diagnosis of a disease to help you stop acting stupidly.

The biggest change I saw in AA and treatment over the years was in what had been the line between "abuse and addiction." It has now been blurred to the point where most new attendees are being told they need treatment for a disease that many/most just don't seem to have—"chemical dependency or alcoholism." This results in many newcomers running for the door as soon as they see what's up.

A Common Description of an Alcoholic

Chronic alcoholics get delirium tremens (DT's), hangovers, and blackouts, and they still cannot stop. Some drink themselves into an alcoholic, brain-damaged condition that causes a permanent mental impairment. They then are no longer able to function as anything like normal. According to 2012 data from the NIAAA.

The lucky ones, if there is such a thing, get institutionalized, diapered, and cared for the rest of their much-shortened lives. Nobody, it seems, recovers from alcohol-brain damage. The rest end up as homeless, living in abandoned buildings, under bridges, etc. I have learned these are among the smallest percentage of drinkers, but they have always been among us. This was however, the major group populating AA in its beginning.

Think about this a moment.

Who in their right mind would want to attend meetings with people like these, much less be seen anywhere else with them? This was no social club as we know AA today.

Only their peers, the other drunks who also had no choice in the matter any longer and nowhere else to go, would want to associate with such AA members. This is why, too, in early AA, members never referred to themselves as being "chemically dependent." They may have been so, but, as I said earlier, they only called themselves drunks.

And lastly, in the 1970s, when I first arrived, nobody outside the doors of any AA club ever talked about the potent combination of caffeine, nicotine, and sugar most of the members were flying on in their meetings (no exaggeration). The conversations in those squads were surely the most spirited ever heard in an AA meeting, and they truly haven't been as enthusiastic since AA went nonsmoking and stopped pushing cookies. However, cookies being served at meetings may now have come back into vogue along with another abusive behavior: **overeating, instead of over-drinking.**

Chapter 10
Starting Over, Again

1976. Louise had had enough; she took our two-year-old baby and left me for a two-bedroom apartment in West St. Paul. We sold the house. I moved on to share a two-bedroom mobile home with an old drinking buddy, Lenny, who had recently, coincidentally, sobered up too. In fact, he was also a former drinking pal of my old friend Greg, who had also quit without the help of AA.

Lenny never did share Sheila with us, however; he wouldn't have anyway—he was gay. Rooming with Len allowed me some needed time to get back on my feet and find a new job. Sharing this smallish house with him and two dogs put a crimp on dating for both of us. We were always respectful of each other, and one or the other would go sleep somewhere else if needed, for some privacy. Most evenings I went to an AA meeting while Lenny cruised the gay bars.

Even with our best intentions, we started to crowd each other. In the spring, I located a nice one-bedroom apartment near my childhood neighborhood called Indian Mounds Park. Having a full-time job now made life a lot easier.

The position was as a job developer and placement specialist for the city, an extension of my AA attendance and my previous sales work. I met a new young lady there, Pam, who worked in a related field with an office nearby. She loved to water ski, and so did I, and her brother owned a ski boat.

There were a lot of fun weekends with Pam and her friends. Drinking was never a problem; they simply didn't drink much. Besides, I was still going to meetings and abstaining from alcohol. I was smitten with Pam. She was beautiful and accomplished, and I always wondered what she saw in me, a nearly middle-aged man with a small son. But we had a great time for the year and a half our relationship lasted.

Looking back, I remember she had an apparently alcoholic father, a very shrewish mother, and a couple of divorced older brothers. She always said she'd never get married. Maybe this said a lot about why I could not get her to be more serious about the two of us together.

A couple of other things probably contributed to the end of the relationship: I really did, at the time, want to be married again, and I was a womanizer who pretty continuously flirted with other women—especially her girlfriends. As brain dead as it sounds, I'd never really noticed how much friction this caused us. After a year and a half, Pam and I went separate ways. Not at all what I was hoping for, and I didn't handle it well emotionally. I had wanted a committed relationship with her, but she could not overlook some of my character issues like the flirting. I asked her if this bothered her and she said, no, she just didn't want to be married.

A couple weeks after the breakup, I had taken the opportunity to date a couple of women "in-house," so to speak. One was an employment center client, Jane, a cute brunette with a very definite twinkle in her green eyes. It just so happened that she too had worked with Pam on getting a vocational school grant. This being completed, Pam herself brought Jane over to introduce to me for placement assistance.

I found Jane a job in her new trade, and I asked her out. We had a nice time together, but she informed me she was not looking for anything serious right now. However, the evening did conclude with our going to bed together. In the following days, I bumped into Jane from time to time around the office, but it never went anywhere past the one encounter.

At about this time, a visiting rep named Sue from an outside agency came in to pick up some files she had called me about. We met in person and I liked her, so I asked her for a date. Very similar results, as with Jane. Maybe not as wild, but Sue was very giving, in an enthusiastic way, just the same.

Some days later, I returned to the office after lunch and was about to turn a corner to enter my work area. This would bring me within ten feet of where Pam, Jane, and Sue were visiting and having a nice laugh. Luckily, they were distracted enough to not notice me, and I did a rapid about-face and got out of there before they did.

This was a unique and unusual experience for me, seeing the three girls who had all recently been lovers of mine, visiting with each other. Very surreal, but it really didn't cheer me much. The way I saw it, I'd had a fling with each of them, but still didn't have anybody of my own—which is what I wanted most of all.

Looking back, I see that I was really immature at this time in my life. All I know for sure is I didn't get over Pam easily. I thought about her constantly, even obsessed about her. I would like to think I'd love someone for the right reasons. But more and more often, looking at the way I handled romance, I was not so sure.

This knowledge was troubling enough, especially if one sees the same negative behavior rearing itself repeatedly. My father had been a flirtatious fellow, and the ladies all seemed to like it; maybe my mother did not, but she never said anything!

So Pam was gone, and try as I might, I couldn't replace her. Further, I was depressed, pissed-off, and dissatisfied with the way my life was going. Whatever the cause, it probably wasn't the best time for me to revisit another old girlfriend—Mary Jane.

Chapter 11
Sobriety Gone, Then Found Again

1978. A new neighbor had moved into my apartment building, a middle-aged hippie named Al, who was a pot-dealer who also dealt in other drugs. Every night when I came home from work, I could smell the burning weed as soon as I entered the hallway of our building.

By the time I had changed clothes, gone for my bike ride, and returned, the marijuana residue was even stronger. Actually, I was surprised the cops driving patrol by the apartment building with their windows down couldn't smell it, too. It was so pungent. It wasn't long before I began buying pot from my neighbor-dealer Al. Did I mention I was depressed? Pot is a very effective depressant.

Shortly after I had reestablished myself with pot, my job with the city ended. After five years. I'd had six or so months of full unemployment benefits to collect and a new compulsion with marijuana to get reacquainted with. I also left AA. I was unencumbered and unrestrained by anything: starting with abstinence, a wife, a girlfriend, a job, shortage of money, time? I'd had it all, for a while. Maybe I even actually looked for a job…well, maybe not.

I was kidding myself—there was no way I was going to kick pot as long as the money held out. And it didn't. One day the unemployment checks ran out, the rent was due, and the first ex-wife was demanding past-due child support payments and had me served by the court.

The wolf was at the door, and I was ill equipped to fight it. I had smoked pot, exclusively, every day for six months. I didn't drink or do any other drugs during this time, just pot. I told my friends that since I hadn't drunk for three years, there was no reason to start now. I did have a beer occasionally. After a while, though, I definitely needed some major cough suppressant medicine—codeine worked very well. I did not get drunk at all during this period—stoned, yes, drunk, no.

I didn't need to get drunk. The pot was ruining what was left of my once excellent health. Although I had smoked regular cigarettes ever since I was a teenager, I had also always worked out with a combination of long bike rides and weightlifting. During the last couple of months, those rides and workouts dwindled to nothing at all. As the Big Book says, "I was licked." Out of desperation, I called my old AA pal Doc, who had by then become something of a big shot himself in our local AA club.

He was a successful dentist, well known in the area, and my friend. Back in both of our early sober days, we used to lunch together at his special table at the Fox, a fancy restaurant. Pam and I had double-dated with him and his girlfriend, Barb. I was frequently invited to his cabin in the Brainerd area, back when life was still good for me.

He was a true friend, and when I told him how much trouble I was in, Doc didn't hesitate to reach out to help. Years earlier, he had come to his first AA meeting at the Summit AA club, which I had moved to from my old Westside group about a year before. And now he was established there, too, doing service work and getting to be known also.

Doc was pretty messed up in those early days. On the one hand, he was a little grandiose, and in the style of the 1970s, he wore a gold double-knit leisure suit and topped off his image by arriving in a new, gold Lincoln Continental Mark V. (He had three ex-wives and three kids too.) He definitely turned some heads—especially susceptible were Barb, his beautiful future wife, and I, again, with my wealth-envy thing going on.

This was about a year after I'd gone to my first AA meeting at the Lake Minnetonka club. For all his bravado and coolness, Doc needed a friend, and I was a good fit. He and I started hanging around together, and soon Pam and Barb joined in.

1981. Doc pulled some strings and found an opening for me at the Twin Town treatment center. Not a minute too soon. I had been evicted from my apartment. I had no money and no friends left I hadn't already hit up. My weight had dropped from 165 to just 138 pounds at check-in, just from smoking pot for six months! I spent twenty-eight days in-patient, then another couple months in a seedy halfway house in South Minneapolis while, especially in treatment, I got reacquainted with "the program."

I got my first sober job as a dishwasher in a local diner. I was thirty-six years old and glad to have found it. A couple weeks later, I upgraded to busboy status at a very nice restaurant in Bloomington. Things were looking up until I came back to the halfway house late one night after work and got into a scuffle with one of the residents there. This guy Donnie had borrowed my Trek bicycle and broken its frame.

I still had anger issues, including one I used to justify punching Donnie in the nose. However, the fact this asshole had started it made no matter to the house management, and we were both evicted.

Are you starting to see how things run in patterns sometimes?

Things can improve too. Now, instead of being penniless, I had some money saved, I had a car (with all of my belongings in it), and my parents were now willing to allow me to stay in their basement until I found a new place. I had a wonderful couple of weeks with Dad while living with him and Mom again.

I helped him build his dream garage in the backyard. It was now springtime and warm. We had to cut down a couple of small maple trees, dig out the foundation trench, and get it ready for the cement finishers to pour the footing.

This was the most continuous quality time Dad and I had spent together in many years. I didn't hunt, fish, shoot archery, or donate endless hours to church-related functions like he did. We lived in two different worlds. I did occasionally have a drink with him in the old days, before I quit, but not lately.

I will always be grateful for the time we had together then.

The next move took me to a beautiful rooming house in old Mahtomedi on the east shore of White Bear Lake. A big old house with a half a dozen sober men and women sharing separate bedrooms and a couple of bathrooms, and the kitchen, living room, etc. It was a fun time, mostly. Some more growing up took place there, but thankfully—no more fistfights.

I also went to barber school, having gotten a grant and a part-time job to help pay for it.

Chapter 12
A New Start, with Ladies Too

1982. I was busy again, and it felt good. I got reacquainted with my son. I had never stopped speaking with TJ on the phone; it was just difficult to see him when I didn't have a car. But it all got taken care of. He was now nine years old, and he loved to come out and stay with me. The house was a short walk to a private beach on the lake, with good fishing and a dock to jump off of and go for a swim.

I was now going to AA meetings at a club in North Oakdale exclusively by now, two to three meetings a week, along with all of my other activities. It wasn't a fancy club by any means, not like the Summit AA or the one at Lake Minnetonka, but it did have a lot of the kind of people I grew up with on the East Side.

I was becoming well known there, too, and got asked to serve on the club's management and volunteer boards. This felt like an honor, but it was sometimes a pain, as there were too many hardheaded egos, with differing points of view. I like to think I had learned something about service work there. My guess is I did; it felt like I was doing what I'd always seen my dad do.

Things were going along rather well, considering all of the demands on my time. Then I met Susie and Debbie, two beautiful, youngish thirty-something-year-old women. I had met each of them at a different AA meeting and had asked Debbie out first and had a wonderful time.

She was soft and sensitive, quiet and good-humored in an understated, ironic way. We went out twice, the second date ending with a wonderful make-out session with a lot of heavy petting. She was also separated but not divorced with two teenaged children and an estranged husband who had a reputation as a kind of a maniacal type who demanded too much of her time.

It may have been selfish of me, but when I found out her husband had a nasty reputation—as much as I liked her—I just didn't feel the urge to put on the knight's armor and attempt to "rescue the maiden," as it were.

Then an event of major proportions occurred in my life.

The other girl, Susie, had set her sights on me from the start, and as her new boyfriend, I quickly discovered my life would never be the same again. We had met when she was dating my housemate, the Rev. Gordy. We called him the Reverend, because as a tall, lean fellow, he wore black everything—all the time—shirts, pants, vests, and boots. He also had slicked-back, black hair and a widow's peak. He looked very ministerial. He didn't play the role, however.

He had taken a massage class somewhere and acquired a portable, folding massage table he took everywhere. He especially made good use of it up in his room, with a seemingly endless stream of young women going up there it seemed daily.

Susie was one his "clients." She has since maintained for decades now that nothing untoward ever took place up there (and I have come to accept it). She was a strawberry blonde, leaning toward red, with a faint spray of freckles across her medium-sized, somewhat Roman nose and the warmest brown eyes I've ever seen.

She was medium height and slender in a nicely curvaceous way, with medium breasts, very round, firm hips, and strong, shapely legs. Where Debbie had been more voluptuous, Susie was very athletic, and I loved her for it. One of her best features has always been her laugh; it sounds like short trumpet bursts and you can hear it for incredible distances, although it's not really loud. It has actually allowed me to locate her at large public gatherings and events. Her laugh is infectious; everyone who's heard it loves how it rings with joy.

We met in the fall of the year I had moved into the Mahtomedi home. We spent a lot of evenings walking the lovely, tree-lined roads bordered by converted summer cottages that gave Mahtomedi an old resort-village appearance, which it is. Since both of us were pretty broke, it was one of our favorite pastimes to stroll up to the local library a mile or so from my home.

Those walks helped us share our life stories and cemented the relationship. We had both, as AA says, "walked the walk and talked the talk," and had a lot of healing to do from each of our own misspent lives.

One evening (we had dated a few times by then), I arrived to pick her up at her home to find her wearing, barely, a wispy pale-green party dress with no back and hardly any front to speak of. She had picked this dress to wear to her friend's wedding reception and, coincidentally, to mention to me (who had no idea about her true age at this time), she was only twenty-four years old—fourteen years my junior!

This was another of those heart-stopping moments in a life filled with more than my share of them. This girl with the looks of a Valkyrie goddess was brimming with sexy, fabulous beauty, and she was all mine, if I would have her.

I'll spare you the suspense; we were not apart again for the next twenty-nine years! This particular evening's activities ended up with my next heavy petting session of the summer.

Up until then, I had been taking it slow with her. It wasn't too many more months before we moved in together. Now in an apartment of our own, I had a real home where I could have my son over to at least spend weekends with me. Half a year later, I passed the state barber boards, and then Susie and I married.

Chapter 13
Sailing through Thirty Years of AA and Changes

2010. The next couple of decades slipped by with hardly any notice of time. Marriage, with no more children beyond my son between us, until he married and had three boys, and then Susie and I had three grandsons.

We both continued to attend weekly AA meetings, sponsoring newcomers, volunteering on club boards, and occasionally speaking at "open meetings" before larger audiences. Susie and I rapidly became the "Barbie and Ken" of local AA.

It was fun for a while; we both liked the notoriety or even fame. After a time, though, we too were taken for granted and didn't miss the popularity when it was gone. Our careers had grown too.

We were so busy we hardly noticed our relationship was seriously coming apart. I do know we tried confronting it: the fights, verbal assaults, resentments later, a serious loss of warm feelings for one another. In the end, though, as always, it was easier to just stay distracted and not talk about it, beyond the blame game, of course. By then, even "the program" couldn't save "us."

Not as if we didn't try; for distraction, I now believe, we were able to eventually buy a home and sailboats, and we had many extended travel vacations. Our favorites were the BVIs and the Florida Keys, wonderful amusements all.

The biggest prize (we thought) was being able to purchase a large sailboat to keep at a marina in the Apostle Islands area of Lake Superior.

Hey, maybe this "envy and lust" thing can work for a person after all. Seriously, though, buying boats was never about keeping up with anyone else. We just loved sailing, and the Apostle Islands National Park is one of the best sailing places in the world and a huge, on-going diversion.

We still had to each bring ourselves along, though.

Sailing among all those primitive islands, with their hills, forests, rocky beaches, and windswept cliffs, many populated with wildlife, including black bear. Each island is within a few miles of other islands, which makes the area a sailor's paradise.

Sailboats are beautiful, graceful, and elegant but not fast. The best of them will not even get to ten miles per hour; the average is more like five to seven. Speedboats will go double and triple that, just so you nonsailors know. However, getting around in a timely manner can be important, especially if stormy weather is blowing in.

Early on in my AA career, I found sailing to be a perfect metaphor in a lot of ways, ever since my friend and AA sponsee, John C., introduced me to it. Sailing is not about instant gratification; it takes effort and concentration, and many things have to work together for you to successfully navigate your craft. Sometimes storms, like other events in our lives, force decisions upon you unexpectedly.

On Lake Superior, this is always a risk. Remember the wreck of the *Edmund Fitzgerald*? She was a famous iron-ore carrier ship that sank in a freak storm in late November. All boaters offshore on Lake Superior think about her.

The Apostle Islands is the kind of place you just want to return to over and over. Being able to go there was one of the rewards of a successful recovery from my pot abuse and always satisfying as well as absorbing.

I have flown over these islands in a small airplane; they are small and large, long or round in shape. They reminded me of homemade cookies cooling on a cooking sheet when I was a small boy.

Located about three hours from our home, the boat is easy to reach for the long weekends we liked so much. Susie and I were usually able to get away early on Friday, which, if we departed by early afternoon, would have us on the boat by dinnertime if the traffic in Duluth didn't slow us up too much.

Upon arrival, we could load our supplies on the boat, untie from the dockage, get our first argument about who was in charge out of our systems, and be under way within minutes.

An easy two- to three-hour sail (after "further discussions"), would have us "dropping the hook," and anchoring in any one of a dozen or more coves or bays, twenty or so miles out.

Leaving the marina was the first part of the adventure. Backing a forty-foot boat out of its snugly fit dockage was like wriggling out of a tight pair of pants, only you're not supposed to make contact with the other boats on your way out.

This was especially challenging while engaged in verbal fisticuffs: "Look out, you're going too fast…"; "Are you watching?"

Once out in the slipway, you shift the motor to forward and try to avoid being pushed by current or wind while steering the watery avenues between other yachts, heading toward a stone, zigzag breakfront to the open water, which, I was continually reminded, I didn't pay enough heed to (maybe not, but I never did touch it).

Equate driving a larger sailboat in a harbor to backing up a school bus on an icy driveway (which I have done). You just sort of point it and hope for the best.

Once in open water, away from the marina, if you are a sailor and there is any useful wind, you will want to rig the sails. Hauling an eight-hundred-square-foot mainsail up a sixty-two-foot mast takes much effort, coordination, *and more negotiation* from all hands. Once done, you can bear off, which allows the wind to catch your sails and start drawing you forward.

Now the magic begins for a sailor. You turn off the rumbly droning of the motor, which then allows the sounds of a sailboat underway to surround you—the splashing of water against the hull accompanied by the whooshing of the wind flowing past the sails.

In heavier weather, the splashing can become banging, and the whooshing turns to howling, but these conditions, while always to be avoided, sometimes are necessary or you cannot get anywhere. The effort of getting there was the reason for the journey in the first place.

A sloop-rigged boat such as ours (one mast, two sails) is a joy under way. Whispering along under wind power alone, heeled over at ten to fifteen degrees and porpoising gently through the waves as they gurgle under the hull. Hours spent like this allow one to achieve a Zen-like state I believe is superior to any artificially created by drugs or alcohol (if one party stops "correcting" the other long enough to enjoy it).

Marina, village, and homes now far behind, the view has changed to miles of open scenic waterscape with more islands and bays coming into view with each passing boat length.

For all the effort we've put forth, we only achieve a modest speed of seven knots or so, which allows a continuously relaxed view of all surrounding us in our journey, providing one of Lake Superior's famous pea-soup fogs hasn't overtaken us. Not this day, the visibility is distinct.

We steer a steady course toward the island we (finally) picked for this evening's anchorage.

We have twelve to fifteen miles to travel, so I steer slightly nearer to the passing shorelines of Basswood and Hermit islands (which I am continually reminded *I am passing much too close to)*. I never touched anything here either, but she has a point.

I would do this (I would have told you), to allow us to view in passing the thick forest above the granite cliffs and rock formations, carved by Lake Superior's famous storms and crashing seas during winter months when the place refreshes itself, sometimes with a vengeance.

Today there is a gentle fifteen-knot breeze and a one- to two-foot sea, almost perfect. One of the other rewards of sailing is getting your craft to cooperate with the weather and sea conditions with enough skill to journey to a destination. Once we have arrived at the island of our choosing, we need to "park the boat." I call to Susie, "Ready to douse the sails?"

"Ready," she replies after we settle on where to put the boat (and she again reminds me of everything about this exercise which I need to do).

An ominous tone usually took over Susie's persona here with this part of the voyage. She'd gone from her cheerful, amiable crewmate self to an ill-tempered deck-chief, barking orders at me in a none-too-friendly tone. What had engendered this cynicism in her?

Dousing the sails entails releasing the halyards (ropes) holding the sails up, and allowing the sails to slide down the mast and relax over the boom-spar and onto the deck. There they must be gathered and lashed down to keep them neat and out of the way and ready again for use when departing.

During this exercise, using the boat's diesel engine, I attempt to keep it on a heading directly into the wind. Once the sails are doused and stowed, the anchor needs to be deployed. A simple matter of selecting a location off of the beach or shoreline, allowing for what is known as a seven to one scope, meaning seven feet of anchor rode out for each one foot of depth. In ten feet of water, you need seventy feet of anchor rode. This practice allows for "swing-room" for the boat in changing wind conditions, as well as extra purchase or bite for the anchor in the event of foul weather or high winds pulling the boat away.

Her mood change would usually pass once the boat was moored.

The boat is now anchored; everyone breathes a sigh of relief and turns their attention to the surrounding scenery. The tree-lined bay protects us on three sides. The sandy beach is lined with a dense forest of primitive growth of birch, pine, oak, maple, and many other species of trees. The undergrowth is so thick as to be almost impenetrable. These islands haven't been logged in almost a century. It's a wilderness.

Anchored nearby on most summer weekends are thirty to forty other boats. Everyone keeps a good space from their neighbor; noise is at a minimum, if at all. There is the occasional friendly hail of a craft recognizing another familiar boat; many spontaneous parties will spring up this evening.

Soon the air is scented with the fragrance of spices and cooking: meats, fish, corn on the cob, and what-have-you. Everyone settles in for a relaxed evening while waiting for dinner to cook. Many will venture ashore using their boats' dinghies to get their land-legs back, hiking.

Soon the sun is setting, first replaced by a multicolored orange to pink twilight and then followed by a velvety blackness, dotted by uncountable thousands of stars. The North Star is quickly located by following the front-pan face of the Big Dipper (Google it).

For the first dozen years Susie and I did this, our beverage-of-choice was nonalcoholic: soda, juice, and coffee, anything *but* beer, wine, or booze. *We would both have told you it didn't matter if we were not drinking.* For us, staying away from the booze, pot or drugs was the price of admission, and we dearly believed it to be so.

I occasionally wondered whether an adult beverage, beer or wine, have calmed the waters? Nah, sadly it was too late for a solution to any of our problems. Finally, we did have the "end of the day" glass of wine on our last sail together—which really was too little, too late.

The other changes to my life also occurred gradually.

The barbering did not last beyond the first three years; standing all day was too hard on my thirty-eight-year-old feet and back. I also believe my ADD kicked frequently, and I spent the next twenty-nine or so years as a sales rep selling life insurance, an automotive technical service, and mortgages, and occasionally driving a limousine.

A pretty typical ADD life, I think, along with, of course, weekly AA meetings—until three years ago when my return to drinking alcohol dictated that I leave AA, for the last time. Thanks to; moderate imbibing, whatever God you believe in, and the wine producers of the world!

Chapter 14
Out the Back Door of AA

The changes, including many I personally witnessed, from early, original AA to today's AA meetings, went like this:

1935. When AA was founded (I wasn't born yet) and through the 1970s, when I first did attend, it was difficult for anyone like me to be accepted into Alcoholics Anonymous (AA), given that I did not meet their qualifications for membership. Meaning, I was not a chronic DT -suffering drunk. I also wasn't hospitalized with liver failure, kidney failure, or any other alcohol-related problems.

I, simply put, frequently drank too much.

In those first AA and Oxford Groupers clubs in the 1930s, there was a serious lack of space for meetings. They were often held in each other's homes. They would just not have wanted me then. Also, the prospects—local drunks they *were* able to work with—were almost exclusively found in jails, in hospitals, or even under bridges.

In contrast to the crowds of drink and/or drug abusers of today, there weren't nearly as many prospects to pick from then. The courts were not ordering them to treatment or to AA wholesale, as would occur in later years. True, the Oxford Groupers and the early AAs were recruiting, but on a much smaller scale than today.

At the time the first edition of the book *Alcoholics Anonymous* was written in 1939, this was the case for the few meeting places existing anywhere. This quickly changed, however, as AA caught on.

When the original text was published, AA stated of itself in the foreword to the first edition of the Big Book, "We, of Alcoholics Anonymous, are more than 100 men and women who have recovered from a seemingly hopeless state of mind and body"!

This passage goes on to conclude with this key sentence: "to show other alcoholics precisely how we have recovered is the main purpose of this book."[1]

This, then, has become one of the great exaggerations or misstatements of the past eighty plus years!

Here's why:

1. *Almost nobody* was staying continually sober! Not then and *not since*! Study after study today shows AA's *initial* recovery numbers are dismal: less than 3 percent![2] But neither AA nor **the treatment industry** ever corrected this point.
2. The problem-drinkers who do keep coming back to "try, try again," *only* make up about a third (31 percent, in AA's own study), of the membership who finally do put some (undocumented) years of sobriety together. Long-term, the numbers fall even more drastically.[3]

If you pool all of this data with a national population of over 310 million here in the United States alone, the sheer number of drunks—*a couple of million claimed*—who do end up going to meetings makes it appear as if AA is succeeding immensely!

However, *the actual AA attendance numbers don't bear this out at all*. The other old-timers I visited with about this topic in recent years have all noticed this continual decline in attendance.

Yes, there is a core group of members at each club, but the vast majority of weekly attendees continually turns over, and new people replace last week's new people.

Older members, from even as little as a few years ago, just aren't there anymore. This group has gone away, and most do not return. However, this phenomenon is hidden in the onslaught of court-ordered newcomers, which makes it appear as if the clubs, if not flourishing, are at least holding their own!

However, study after study shows they are not.

Note: The former regular attendees have also been replaced by the newbies streaming through the "revolving door." If this were not so, the clubs would still be growing noticeably and they truly are not.

AA's population has been static since the mid-1990s, even with continually strong referral numbers from the courts and treatment centers.

From 1939, with the first publication of the Big Book, through about 1990, AA certainly did spread. There had never been anything like this recovery and treatment program for alcoholics and addicts on such a grand scale. It looked great too.

1970. The "open door" to AA that replaced the rigid, previous requirements for membership made for standing room only for a time in the clubrooms at the rapidly expanding AA movement of those years. The growth in membership has long since leveled off. Early AA had grown on its own, with the limited help of hospitals and the courts, but by the end of the 1960s, the treatment center industry was flourishing. As with any new business, this treatment thing desperately needed to show a profit.

This new concept of treatment centers, I noticed, had, over the years, given the AA clubs a whole new face.

This was not the former face of burned out, haggard drunks we had come to associate with the concept of being an alcoholic at the downtown clubs of the world. No sir (or madam). The inpatient or new, outpatient treatment programs sent huge numbers of their graduates, as they called them, to AA. As a result, the membership began to look more and more like the rest of us; they were becoming us!

There certainly were a lot of prospects out there. We all knew of someone who was likely a drunk or problem drinker. Their spouses, their employers, the cops who arrested them, and the judges who sentenced them sure did. But, I often wondered, did they all really need treatment?

Some had been charged with a DUI only once or twice, not exactly a "pattern of abuse." Again, I observed, it seemed as if the **treatment centers** were trying to keep a lot of beds in a lot of chemical dependency wards full. This treatment thing was big, and it seemed to be high profit too. Put the patients in beds, give some nursing and counseling care, and feed them is about all there is needed—for most—at $1000 a day! Adding to this profit margin is the free, no-cost aftercare and follow-up, thanks to us all at AA!

I don't remember anyone asking us for our "treatment center" counseling certificates at AA; they just kept referring patients to us anyway.

All of which begs another question: namely, where is the priority here? Is it to first identify and then treat drunks and addicts, or is it just to fill beds?

A lot of these prospects did not qualify for or did not have insurance coverage for treatment, so, instead they were referred directly to AA with these consoling words: "don't worry if you couldn't get into treatment; the founders of AA didn't have any treatment to go to, either, and they still recovered!"

I really saw this firsthand at my meetings. There were a lot of the newcomers who said they had been washed out of treatment and told to go to AA, which they did try. Even if they managed to sit through an entire first meeting, many, most would not return.

As I observed, since the **treatment centers** seem to have all the money, always remember the golden rule: "whoever has the gold gets to make the rules"! AA's new rule, from their friends at the **treatment centers**, was "no more rules"!

2011. As I stated in chapter 3, the next biggest change in the past thirty years of my life, because during which time I had been abstinate in AA, was to return to "social drinking."

I had unintentionally been conducting a personal experiment about intoxication for the past three years. During that time, I had needed to have several surgeries and several dental procedures, each of which required me to be anesthetized and given prescription pain medication later by my doctors.

These were operations such as root canals, a nasoplasty, and a foot and then a hand surgery, each one needing several weeks to a month or more of recovery. They were all performed within months of each other, and each had quite painful recoveries.

The results left me with quite a collection of painkillers: Vicodin, Percocet, and Tramadol, etc. When I say collection, I mean as many as several bottles of each of these to be found sitting in the back of my medicine cabinet, each unused for many weeks or months.

These had been prescribed to me by my doctors at each procedure, and when, after the healing began, I no longer needed help for the pain, I had stopped taking them!

The pain had subsided; I had healed, and even though I occasionally enjoyed the buzzy feeling these pills gave, I had simply stopped using them when pain relief was no longer needed.

What, you may ask, has this to do with socially drinking alcohol? Answer: *It turns out this was an unplanned experiment.* That is, I could not have anticipated this series of medical procedures, in a brief period; it was all just a coincidence!

Note: This ability to take or leave these prescribed narcotics, I am well aware, is where I part company with a lot of my former AA mates. I have believed for many years that getting a feeling of intoxication—of being "high"—is like getting a buzz, and a buzz is a buzz is a buzz. Prescription pain relievers, while always pleasantly effective, have often caused a hang-over effect for me. Not a pleasant one.

Whether the cause of the buzz was the prescribed medicine I'd been using or a glass of wine I'd indulged in, in my experience, usually there was very little difference in the effect.

What I had observed from my experiences over these past years is I could indeed *get a buzz from the painkillers,* and still not lose control or allow an obsession about it to take over my life.

When Susie made her drinking admission to me, years ago, she agreed this had been the case with her too. We talked about it at some length, as you can imagine, I finally admitted to her my own little secret (which I had been keeping especially since my recent sixty-Fifth birthday), which was that I too had concluded that I just might be able to drink socially.

She surprised me by saying, "Yeah, I think you can too; you do live a controlled, moderate life in every other area."

So, after thirty years, I'm now out the back door of AA.

This new pattern of moderate, managed drinking continued for weeks, months, and then years after the first episode without me ever increasing my consumption or losing control.

It continues to this day.

Note: I have also concluded that I must practice moderation in every other area of my life: how much food, especially desserts and other high carbohydrates I eat; how fast I drive my car; how much time I spend watching TV and scanning the Internet; and many other areas as well.

The simple facts are these: I no longer have a weight problem—I was forty pounds too heavy at one time, but lost the excess weight with a low carb diet. (I learned **how** to eat.) I am still slender and haven't received a speeding citation in decades—luck may have had a little to do with this, but not all of it.

Moderation and self-control is what always matters in a successful life. It is essential!

"Social Drinking and AA Don't Mix."

My weekly attendance at AA meetings needed to cease *because of my returning to drinking alcohol.* AA does not endorse any sort of social drinking, especially among its formerly abstinent members. And yet, as discussed above, AA has no problem whatsoever with its members getting a "buzz" from prescription "anti-depressant", and other medications.

I knew, too, that if I did not say anything about my drinking at my meetings, nobody would have any reason to question it, or, subsequently, to ask me to leave, until and if, I returned to being abstinent. But I no longer had a reason to keep my drinking a secret. The main reason I had gone to those meetings in the first place was *not* to not drink alcohol, but primarily *to stop smoking pot!*

Note here also that AA has *no graduation program*—none. There is only your "continued rehabilitation" at weekly meetings or you just leave (in disgrace or silence). How sad. A member spends years, sometimes decades, rehabilitating him- or herself first and then helping scores of others and then after a while, decides to leave.

What thanks is there? The implied message is "Gee, thanks for all your years of selfless service, now get the hell out of here and don't let anyone see you leave."

It doesn't matter how long you had been doing the steps in your meetings, seemingly forever, selflessly sponsoring struggling newcomers, conducting the meetings yourself—you just aren't allowed to leave with any honor.

And just as it was when I had committed to living the sober, AA-prescribed life, I was now committed to living a new, but nonetheless, still accountable lifestyle including the social drinking of adult beverages.

Let me restate this.

I am now committed to living a new, *responsible lifestyle* that includes the social drinking of adult beverages. Just like a large majority of the adult population of the world. I have no regrets about either having been part of or leaving AA.

It was just time to move on.

I've noticed, after several years now of social drinking, I prefer wine and beer. Although I did have the occasional cocktail or highball at first, I found them a little too intense for comfort, so I *choose to limit* the amount I drink, each and (so far), every time.

I do not get drunk, period.

I would also like to tell you how much I really enjoyed the experience of sharing an evening drink with Susie. However, another warning sign I hadn't seen or maybe had chosen not to notice was that she was again spending more and more time away. I wasn't as if I minded this; she did have a life of her own, apart from me. I just didn't realize how separate our two lives had become.

Chapter 15
My Perfect Storm

2011. Spring had finally come, and with it all of the distractions it brings to the denizens of the northern part of America, and specifically, to Minnesota, where I live. I especially welcomed all of the outdoor activities Susie and I both enjoyed so much. I was so caught up in sailing, biking, grilling, etc. that I didn't see it coming—her leaving—I really didn't see it at all.

I had not attended any AA meetings since my March drinking epiphany, and, quite frankly, didn't feel any need to. So, I guess, since I wasn't talking to anyone there (in AA) about our break-up, was I therefore not thinking about it? I don't know the answer.

A lawsuit against our mortgage holder, their clerk had mistakenly listed us as delinquent, from almost 4 years ago had pressed on; we finally got a hearing in April with the mortgage company attorneys. Both sides got to state their cases before the hearing officer, at which time we thought the matter was finally settled.

The mortgage company had admitted their fault in the matter and had stated so for the record! They also said they would make a settlement offer to us in a week or two! We foolishly thought this was finally concluded. This was not to be so.

More months went by without our hearing anything from the attorneys again until June, when the mortgage company announced that its company had been restructured and changed its name. Can you believe it? The company changed its name and thus got another extension! Somehow, this let the company back out of the offer it had agreed to back in April.

In other words, we were back to square one, facing foreclosure.

Also, my employment situation had not improved; in fact, it had worsened. I was still going into the office three or four days a week, but there was less and less to do. Soon I was told my presence wasn't needed; there just wasn't enough work.

I still had not gotten drunk, not once. There had been a rare occasion when I'd had three drinks instead of one or two, and I had discovered I didn't much like the feeling from this many drinks at a time, even if it was only beer or wine. So I avoided doing more than two. Just order a side of water, and you will always have something to sip on.

Also, I knew drinking oneself into oblivion would not cure any of these problems. I had seen enough of what excessive drinking will do to a person and did not wish to indulge.

Then came the day in early August when I arrived home from my Wednesday business networking lunch. Coincidentally, it was the same day Susie was planning on leaving for a long weekend with some girlfriends, I thought.

She was sitting at the kitchen lunch counter when I arrived in a cheerful mood and asked her how she was doing.

She said, "Fine, but I'm leaving you again!"

I felt as though she had hit me in the testicles with a baseball bat. The blood rushed to my head, and I had to sit down. She said, "I can't talk now. I have to get ready and leave."

I was too stunned to reply.

Within minutes, she was gone and I was left there with the most desperate feeling I have had maybe in my whole life. I had no one to talk to, to talk to about it. A lesser man, I'd like to think, would've done something outrageous at this time, like getting drunk!

I was honestly too depressed to get drunk! All I knew was my world was crashing down around me, and all I wanted to do about it was go to sleep and hopefully never wake up.

So I lay down for a nap.

I found no comfort there because the dreams kept waking me up: dreams of being homeless, unemployed, and broke, and now (almost) sixty-five years old. Oh, and let's not forget being alone—especially being alone.

This all-together, brought about a desperation that further muddled all reasoning.

I seriously challenged myself here about whether or not I still loved her. I know it doesn't make sense, as I still felt I did, but I was so panicked and discouraged about everything else, it was the first thing I thought of. Obviously, she had left for a reason. I had been in a terrible slump for a long time, more than a year. I had not been good company a lot of this time.

I thought I still loved her and probably always would (wrong, I finally outgrew it). I sure wasn't happy with her, even if I understood why she'd left me. If the situations were reversed and I had been she, I might have left too, maybe even sooner! I had been stuck in a rut, and nothing I had tried to do to change was working. But now, I really was depressed. A good thing I didn't know "the rest of the story," which was that she had left me to go visit a new boyfriend out on the East Coast, "where her girlfriends lived."

Maybe it's just my now-cynical outlook on this whole episode, but she seemed to look awfully pert and "done-up" to go visit the girls. Oh well, the memory affects what one wants to recall, and I have no pleasant recollections about this matter at all.

As Mick Jagger once sang, "…you know I used to love her, but it's all over now."

As luck would have it, I had a doctor appointment the next day for my annual physical and decided to use the opportunity to ask about some depression medication. My doctor asked me if I would like her to administer a simple quiz they use to determine if an individual is depressed. I said yes.

The quiz was eleven questions about depression and anxiety. I answered ten in the affirmative. The doctor said, "You're depressed, all right." She prescribed an antidepressant immediately. I also asked her about getting some counseling help, and she agreed to this also.

I slept a lot for the first couple of weeks. Gradually I returned to working every day and soon had a new position as an appointment setter and data entry clerk for a local heating company. Within a few weeks, I was somewhat closer to feeling normal, with fewer anxiety attacks, better sleep, and so on, than I'd felt in months.

I really didn't know which had helped me the most, being able to work more regularly or taking the antidepressants, but I was feeling better. I had a glass of wine most evenings, even though I know mixing drugs and alcohol is a dangerous practice, but I kept it under control. The diet again.

Eventually, with the doctor's help, I weaned myself off of the antidepressants, but I continued to see a psychologist for a few more months. I am also happy to report I still didn't get drunk over this or anything else.

I did not go back to AA either.

I'd had my "acid test" and passed! That is, I proved to myself I can live in an adult world that may include social, relaxed drinking, even (especially) in a crisis!

The point that seemed ever more clear to me was how in control I would have to become over all of my personal life choices, no matter what external forces were bringing on to me. If it is raining, you can choose to wear a raincoat. You don't have to; you could go without one and get wet. You can also choose whether to wear a hat or not; have breakfast or not; take your car or walk; drive sensibly or speed and drive recklessly. The decisions we make every day are endless.

I realized again and again that I am not some helpless victim.

Choices, choices—they never let up. Most of them we just make without thinking. To me, it is the blessing and the curse of having a "free will." And because of it, as long as we live, the choices never end, provided we still have control of our faculties. So my journey continues, and so does, hopefully, personal progress along with it.

Big setback: this first winter, in January, I fell in an icy parking lot and tore the rotator cuff in my shoulder. So, I had another surgery, followed by many months of painful recovery and more prescription pain medication. I spent months, often alone, wearing a brace. Sleepless nights sometimes spent walking the frozen, even stormy streets of my neighborhood to ward off the anxiety I had awoken with at 3:00 in the morning. Occasionally treating myself to a (microwaved) egg, ham, and cheese muffin with a glass of cabernet which helped immensely.

These were literally some of the longest and darkest days I have spent in my life. It was almost a daily struggle for me to survive physically and emotionally.

As soon as I was able, I went back to the gym one, then two or three, times a week. I am now there four times! Early on, I joined a card players' club and played several evenings a week, I also took up swing dancing. I had to! Anything less and I might have caved in. The thought of "giving up" haunted me constantly those months.

Did these gym card and dance get-togethers replace my AA meetings?

Absolutely! For social me, regular human contact is a balm, an affirmation of my existence. Since I was no longer employed, it became essential to have the contact with others. What was it that got me "over the hump" and "out of the hole" I'd found myself in?

Grandkids!

I have known of individuals who "cashed in their chips" by committing suicide. I would not leave this legacy to those children. They like me and look up to me. They deserve me at my best.

So, as I had learned so well "in the program," I sucked it up and kept on sucking it up. Eventually, I got through it. I also started swing-dancing lessons, hiking, even dating. I went out with groups of "Meetups"[1] (a social networking group) whom I'd met playing cards. And so there I got to know one particularly special woman.

Two years later. Susie and I are now divorced. She has been living with a new fellow for more than a year. They met at one of the jobs she'd had while we were married. I guess they always liked each other. I wish them well.

One evening at the conclusion of a dance class I'd been attending, while bending over untying my shoes, a small shadow cast itself over me and announced; "you didn't dance with me this evening". Looking up I saw a pixyish lady with brunette hair standing with hands authorativly on hips. Pulling out a chair I asked if she would like to sit down. She did and just like that I had a new girlfriend.

I'll just call her MJ. We have dated for a year. I asked her to marry me, and she accepted. We are still living in separate residences, but that will change soon. We plan to sell both of our houses and get into one of our own.

I had dated a few other women in the past two years; many of them were Susie's age, which was fourteen years younger than me. I am now nearly sixty-nine years old (young), and I have discovered, to my credit that I don't have enough in common with women so much younger any more.

Shortly after meeting MJ, I found out she is less than three years younger than me. This experience was quite a shock, kind of like going through a fourteen-year "time-warp."
This has been mostly pleasant, closing the age gap between me and the lady-love of my life.

Realizing that I had been living in a fantasy world the last twenty years or more with Susie—*a much younger wife does allow one to pretend you are the same age*. It became burdensome and wearying, but it went along with living in a figment of my own imagination.

Along with MJ's maturity comes gentleness and kindness and a patience and wisdom that I just find irresistible to be around. Most of all, she is honest with me.

Susie hadn't been honest with me for a long time.

Years ago, after fighting about it endlessly, she took over our household finances. Her logic was that since she made more money than I did, she should decide how it was spent (Golden Rule, again). As much as I had disagreed with her, since we were both usually very "type A" personalities in matters like this, it became easier for me to just give in.

As time went by, she gained more control over everything financial in our lives. She, however, had no head for planning or finances.

So it was, by the time she had left me, our retirement savings had been picked clean to "pay the bills," as she said. I mostly believed her, however:

She would never discuss with me how to restructure our finances; she just eventually cleaned out our accounts.

I have now had two years to think about this, as I have put my life together again, and I have an interesting supposition to share!

In "the program," one of the many axioms we lived by was "We thought we could find an easier, softer way. (But we could not)"![4] This is just human nature speaking; of course we will take the path of least resistance.

I had been doing so in these matters for years.

The price I personally paid for my acquiescence was this: since I was making less money than she was (which she badgered me about continually), in her eyes, I was therefore the problem here, not her!

Chapter 16
Is AA the Only Way?

2014. The other night I was surfing my TV channels for anything of interest, and a C-SPAN listing had the words *addiction treatment* in its program description. So I gave a look.

The program featured a discussion of the book *"Anatomy of Addiction"*, by its author, Howard Markel, who, it turns out, is a leading expert in addiction treatment (one of the good things to come out of the treatment center expansion, by the way). He stated in this TV interview: "The insidious thing about addiction to mood-altering substances such as drugs and alcohol is you have no way of knowing if you will become an addict, until it's too late"!

I thought about Lefty B's story as Mr. Markel continued with an interesting, though contrary, thesis:

"There are, however, many more people who have used cocaine, speed, all forms of alcohol, etc., and *never become addicted*; then, *there are of those who did.*"

He went on, "Some may even go through withdrawal symptoms, *but they end up able to walk away from it without any further problems.*"

Markel's comments resonated with me. Until hearing them, I had intended this, my book, to be much more of a direct criticism of Alcoholics Anonymous and the treatment center industry.

I don't know how many people will get an opportunity to read my book. I am sure not as many as will read Doctor Markel's; my impact is uncertain at best. Instead of the "weapon of righteousness" my book may have started out as, it has now given way to a *pointed commentary* on AA and addiction treatment from an insider with much accumulated experience to draw from. So I will restate my argument thusly:

While AA is one of several means or paths to recovery...

It is not the only one, and for a surprising number of people, after a time, it ceases to be effective.

AA was created to help what, again?

To help "drunks" (key word here) recover from, as AA describes it, "Alcoholism, a fatal disease of the mind and body."[1] I know the drill well, after spending over half of my adult life attending literally thousands of weekly AA twelve-step meetings.

Do I feel that everyone I sat with in meetings was really an Alcoholic? Of course not, not all of them. The dozens I got to know personally, out of the thousands I attended AA with, were a mix of desperate or depressed people, most of whom abused alcohol and other drugs too.

Many were seriously heavy users who needed to be jailed or court-ordered to treatment where they could be detoxed or hospitalized until they got the drugs out of their bodies so they didn't go into withdrawal, which can bring on seizures or even heart failure and death.

In my opinion, those who make up most of the AA membership today do not drink themselves into the homeless, brain-damaged condition the old-timers and the founders of AA described. Not even close.

What were we all doing there then, *pretending* to be getting cured?

In my own case: AA gave me a structure I needed to deal with my ADD. Also, it had become my exclusive club, complete with its own meeting rooms and rules for attendance. My best friends were there. Luckily, too, "the people we didn't like" either had to 'toe the line' or *get out* (if we really didn't like them)!

This happens, unruly guests frequently show up at AA, often with the repeat court-ordered offenders. But, they would then find another AA group to get their "court cards" signed, either in another room down the hall or better still, in another AA club elsewhere in town. Most clubs do find a way to exclude the people they don't like, troublemakers, etc., which they encounter.

In not a small way, AA is one of the most exclusive clubs in town and sort of socially repressive. For example, you cannot drink alcohol or use any other mood-altering drugs recreationally while attending (talk about a buzzkill), unless the drugs are *prescribed by a physician* (of course).

Some members may, however, continue to use their substance of choice while attending meetings, with the caveat *"If you continue to show that you are making an effort to quit!"* You know, keep on using and yet going to AA meetings. This tactic is difficult to maintain over the long haul, but I have seen it done.

Take the case of Marvin, a charming, seventy-plus-year-old fellow, who owned a successful paint/home decorating store. Marvin had attended meetings at the Summit Avenue AA club. Everybody who met him loved him. Marv had a gift for charming people. He was a regular at the meetings there and always spoke well for himself.

He'd "slipped" (drinking again and getting caught at it, usually with a DUI) a few times, we all knew, but he always came back with just the right amount of contrition, and we were thrilled he chose us again. This went on for years, his slipping thing. Along the way, he sponsored other men, attended the club's social get-togethers, and even served on the AA club's volunteer board of directors.

One sad day, Marvin had a heart attack and died. At the funeral service, his widow, who had remained quite secluded from his AA pals, finally visited with some of us. It's not unusual for many spouses/life partners to never catch on to the AA way of life or to never join the codependency program known as Al-Anon, either.

Whatever her reasons are not important here. She had been known by a few of Marvin's pals, and on the occasion of his funeral, was finally able to unburden herself of this secret of his she had kept these many years, which was this: her Marvin had not ever been a continuously sober man!

Truth be told, she'd said, he'd usually had a martini or highball when he returned home from AA. Why on earth would he do this? He had simply fallen in love with the meetings and the people there, generating more than a few new customers for his store, too. So he'd had a little secret from us after all. I will always have fond memories of him and will always wonder, too, how many other Marvin's are out there, merrily attending AA meetings and then having a drink or two later on for their own reasons.

Note: Just as with situational *alcohol abuse*, there is a risk this too could cause fatal consequences to you or someone else. It is also well known that not everyone who has had an *alcohol-induced episode (gets drunk)* is necessarily an alcoholic. Certainly most, by a large margin, *are not and never will be*.

The same argument can be made about many other activities as well. Some of the many things that could be fatal to indulge in include the following:

- talking or texting on a cell phone while driving, or just distracted driving
- residing in, or even just visiting, some neighborhoods
- chronically speeding while driving, running red lights, swerving, simply talking with anyone while driving
- jaywalking
- auto or motorcycle racing
- participating in dangerous and physical contact sports
- owning a firearm for hunting, sport or personal protection
- overeating and not getting enough exercise
- sexual impulses, for God's sake!

The list is endless.

The thoughtful and skeptical among you might now criticize me by saying "Those things aren't relevant to this discussion," and you'd be correct, sort of...

There is, however, the very valid argument that fatal drunken behavior, driving and otherwise, cannot be taken seriously enough, as Doctor Markel said. And alcoholism of the type that AA was created to treat often does kill people and ruin other lives as well.

Yet isn't that also true about "episodic drunkenness?" Drunk driving is always irresponsible, whether you are a "practicing alcoholic" or just a drunk driver. But, as I said, drunk driving is not alone in this area of fatal consequences. Every day the news is littered with stories of victims of hunting, boating, wilderness camping, and other accidents. People fall down stairs, choke to death at dinner, and get killed by jealous or angry spouses and lovers.

A sage person once said, "The appointment that everyone has someday with the Grim Reaper, the Angel of Death, is one we are never late for."

Life can be dangerous, even if you do try to be cautious.

Chapter 17
Why Bother to Write This Book?

First, the subtitle is very telling. My ex-wife, Susie, suggested it when I told her of my compulsion to tell my story of how I had spent years in AA but then found a way to successfully live without it and remain a responsible, growing, thriving adult.

Because I am no longer welcome at my old Wednesday-night AA twelve-step meeting, which I had attended for the past dozen years (the gossip ran amok upon my leaving, I was told), Susie suggested that I should call it *In the front door, then out the back door of AA*. I almost did, but *Beyond AA* tells the same message, to me.

And so begins my new journey in life.

Truth be told, AA has no place for *graduates* (a backslider, they would call me) anywhere in its closed meetings. Since I have resigned from "The Club," many of my old AA contacts have treated me as a pariah. A few good friends stayed close to me (and for a time, monitored my every move). My old sponsor and sailing partner, John C, is still a friend. This is a good thing, and I know my friends care for me and I am grateful for their support.

Those of you who are uninitiated to the AA rules and culture as well, have to understand one key point to validate my story, which is this: unlike diets, physical therapy, Weight Watchers, and other self-help organizations, AA, does not have any program to help one simply "maintain." There is no achievement of your desired goal and then getting an aftercare plan of how to drink moderately and successfully. (There *is* a way to do this, a diet to follow when drinking; more about this later).

For AA, you are either in or you are out; there just isn't anything else.

And so, after more than thirty years (since 1975 at Beverly Hills AA), I no longer have a membership in what had become a combination of my club, my support group, my friends, and my religion. AA was all of this and more. Besides the many friends I had within the organization, there were also the men I was honored to sponsor, to help them find their way to a successful, sometimes even sober life. Sponsoring and friendships were the most rewarding parts of belonging to AA.

"AA is not the only way"

My biggest issue with AA came to be its implication that IT is the *only thing* that works for the recovery from alcoholism or chemical dependency.

Not true— as shown by my own and other's experiences."

Based on my over thirty years of regular, continuous attendance, I know that this is simply not so in all cases or for all individuals who come to AA meetings looking for help.

It is a solution for many people who had alcohol or chemical dependency problems, however.

AA is fairly good at what it does, but about 90+ percent of the time, it just does not, cannot do all that it claims.

I have had a disconnect with AA about its imperiousness ("rarely have we seen a person fail…") for years, but I kept going to meetings for the above reasons, friendships, life guidance, ADD, etc. And as it is often said there, "If it works, don't fix it."

Again, if you are currently an AA attendee and enjoy the fellowship and the topics discussed at AA meetings, let me say that you are a fortunate individual, and these meetings may be a great benefit to you. Besides the friendships and sponsorships formed there, there can be some much-needed bonding for the newcomers.

I was privileged to be a sponsor for dozens of such men. It was while I was acting as a sponsor that I began to suspect that many of these people who were being encouraged to call themselves "alcoholics" actually were not.

I will attempt to throw light upon this next.

Chapter 18
In Defense of AA, but Also of the 90+ Percent Who Cannot, Will Not Fit-in There

2014. Where do I get the figure of 90+ percent?[1] The experience I had while attending AA meetings as well as the research I've done since I've graduated have shown me that most AA members *were not alcoholics in the traditional AA sense.* In my humble opinion, they were abusers, who, for the sake of harmony within the AA meeting, called themselves alcoholics, addicts, or more likely chemically dependent.

Another example of this type of member: one of my favorite sponsees; Scotty, who came to my Friday meetings at 6:00 p.m. some years ago. He was court-ordered to attend because of two consecutive DUI (driving under the influence) citations.

My first impression of him: a likable guy in his forties, divorced with two young children, a meat cutter by trade, and he was very social. He liked to hang around after the meeting and often would go out to dinner with us, a regular activity. He had an especially good sense of humor and was very personable; he got along with everyone, loved his kids, had a darling girlfriend, and had a good, long-time job he liked where they seemed to like him too.

So what's wrong with this picture?

Answer: he did not, over the year I knew him, show any evidence of alcoholic or chemically dependent behavior, save the two times he was caught driving under the influence. Pretty bad, stupid for sure, but do two DUIs make him an alcoholic?

Maybe not.

The assumption that he was an alcoholic was OK in the beginning of his relationship with AA, which he was court-ordered to attend. And even though he may have protested his conviction, he may well have had either a drinking problem or a serious lack of self-restraint. Both were something I could relate to. With newbies like Scott, I always had this in mind when I first visited with them.

My relationship with a new attendee would typically begin with us getting to know each other during the AA meetings, by listening to each other speak there. Some would go out of their way to introduce themselves. Those were often the court-ordered ones. They would need to get their activity cards signed for their POs (parole officers) for mandatory (mandatory to the "church" of AA?) meeting attendance. To say that they were not happy to be there is an understatement, although a few were relieved that the downward spiral their lives were on might be arrested.

Many old-timers, however, believed 99 percent of new attendees deserved to be there. But in my humble opinion, a long-term jail sentence would be far better and more consequential for many. Most of us got to AA through jail or a court order. Few just walked in.

There were also the really down-and-out ones who, at first, would linger in the back of the room, trying to decide if this time they could really mean it and would be able to quit drinking themselves to death. Some may, but for most of these new attendees, the answer was; probably not. After all, 70+ percent would not continue in *"the program"*.

You could see the look of resignation in their eyes. I would try to see these were looked after, got them a cup of coffee and cookies and, to a newcomer's meeting, and got them the newcomers' package of AA literature for help.

"I am responsible for the effort, not the outcome."[2]

Back to Scotty, who, from the start, was Mr. Charm and good humored and happened to sit in on my meeting. We said hi and became friends. Just like that. Eventually I learned his story; everyone tells their story… if they keep coming, of course. His was not unusual; he drank two to four beers (read a six-pack) almost every day and mainly kept to beer. He had an active relationship with his children and his girlfriend. He got to work on time every day too.

Scotty also claimed he'd had no other alcohol or drug abuse issues. No arrests, health issues, employer warnings to stop drinking, family counselors telling him to quit, etc. He'd just stupidly gotten arrested for DUI two separate times.

One sees a lot of this pattern in AA. That is, in every other area of his life I could see, his drinking, while cumbersome, was almost a nonfactor. So, of course, everybody in the group treated him as if he was a classic alcoholic who would certainly die drunk if he didn't take up our cause and follow us in the twelve steps.

Scott always seemed bemused by this treatment, but, being court-ordered, he went along with it. He asked me to be his sponsor, and so as I always did, I told him my requirements.

Note: Over the years, I came to hate wasting my time sponsoring men (never women) who didn't take this AA stuff seriously. They lied to you, tried to borrow money, asked you to fraudulently sign off on their activity cards, and more. So I created some conditions that had to agree to in order to meet with me.

If I was to work with him, the man I sponsored agreed to do the following:
- He would talk on the phone with me, at least every other day, in the beginning.
- He would have coffee with me, at least once a week, this was aside from the AA meetings.
- He would have to read and discuss with me the first five chapters of the Big Book of Alcoholics Anonymous.
- I would then help him to write his Fourth Step: "We made a searching and fearless moral inventory of ourselves."[3] After which...
- I would listen to his Fifth Step: "Admitted to God, to ourselves and to another human being [in his case, this would be me], the exact nature of our wrongs."[3] In other words, I would "hear his confession," topically, of course.

Since leaving AA, hearing Fifth steps is one of the events I've missed the most. I understand that most religions have a confession procedure. I believe this to be an eye-opening, revealing, and therapeutic action.

The individual gets to more-clearly see, maybe for the first time, the damage his behavior caused. It is an unwritten, not ordered, time-honored tradition for an AA sponsor to hear the Fifth step.

The treatment industry, in its zeal to, I came to believe, "appear relevant" in this matter, has diluted this tradition of AA members looking after their own. More about this later.

Chapter 5 in the Big Book, pages 64 and 65, outlines an *almost too simple* format of how to prepare for a Fifth step. It is so simple that over the years, I believe many of the people I listened to in meetings didn't understand it, and so they ignored it. Or, more likely, they had had one done in a **treatment center** using the "deep psychological" profile format that the **treatment center** had tailored for their chemically dependent patients.

This is OK, as far as it goes. I went to treatment at my second attempt at recovery, the one that lasted twenty-nine years. Treatment helped me to get at some troubling matters that had weighed me down. *If it works, don't fix it...* right? But not everyone gets to go to treatment, and even if you do, the **treatment center's** Fifth step guide, as it's also called, misses a vital point, which I discovered years later. It came to me like this:

Many AA clubs have an "open meeting" format, which entertains larger audiences of recovering people along with their friends, families, drop-ins, and anyone else who wants to attend. While attending one of these, years ago, I heard an AA speaker who told us that the founders and original members of AA took each other's Fifth steps!

This was almost thirty years ago.

There was an almost audible gasp among the hundreds in the hall that evening. We were all thinking the same thing: "We can't do that, we are not trained professionals, therefore not qualified to interpret the 'deep psychological' profile of a Fifth step."

This was because of what we'd been told by the **treatment centers** for the past twenty-plus years. So it had become something of a colloquialism within AA meetings to say, "I did my Fifth step in treatment."

To properly hear a Fifth step (we thought), one needs to be a psychiatrist, certified chemical-dependency counselor, MD (or any other type of doctor, really), priest, clergy, or judge—well, you get the idea.

The **treatment center** administrators knew decades ago, in their beginning efforts, that they had to specialize—meaning that the AA Fifth step, which had been a tried-and-true, effective help for the suffering alcoholic for decades, had to be taken out of the hands of these *so-called amateurs*. This allowed them to create the Fifth step guide pamphlet, which we then came to know as one of the specialties of **treatment centers**.

Back to Scotty.

After I had listened to his Fifth step (which, by now, I had heard from dozens of others), I knew him a lot better. And I must say, when he began to beg off on attending our weekly AA meeting, I wasn't surprised. My old friend and sponsee, John C., asked me one day, "What's the matter with Scott? Why isn't he coming to meetings anymore?"

"I don't think he was an alcoholic," I said.

"How can you say that? Just because he quit us doesn't mean he'll return to drinking, does it?" John replied.

I couldn't tell John what I knew of Scotty because of our AA confidentiality agreement, the anonymous part of AA. But I had observed that our mutual friend just didn't seem to have the character defects and shortcomings described in the Big Book, which are the drinking and drug-use behavior problems of an addict, period.

I have since run across Scotty several times over the years, and he is always glad to see me—at a distance. I suspect he was just afraid I'd try to wrangle him back into AA. And he should have been.

At one time, I would have.

Chapter 19
AA and Emotional Breakdowns

In spite of what I've said so far, please don't think I'm accusing the **treatment center** industry of not being effective. I know it has helped millions of patients and their families. My problem with the industry is this: it gathers in its fish with too wide a net. Is the big profit motive causing all of this?

Of course.

One of my closest AA friends, the other Howard C., had an emotional breakdown over ten years ago. At the time he had been working under a lot of pressure for many months; he always seemed to take his work too seriously, some of us thought.

One evening, in his home, he'd just let it all hang out. He yelled a lot of profanity, very loudly, he threw some knickknacks at the walls, and he couldn't or wouldn't shut up or calm down when his wife asked him to. So, she did the only thing she could think of: *she called the police and had him hauled out of his own house in handcuffs.* (Seriously, I would have left her for that episode, knowing her as I do.)

Well, if he thought he was depressed before this, how was he doing now? Not too well. She'd gotten him committed to a mentally disturbed ward at a state hospital for people like him (angry nut cases), where he spent the next thirty days ruminating over his sins and misdeeds, while attending many group-therapy sessions. Eventually he calmed down.

Note: group therapy doesn't cure you of anything, it just simply allows you to see, compared to at least several other nut cases in your group, that you may not be doing too badly after all. Compared to them, of course.

You will still have to deal with the real world someday, but as I mentioned, they have pills to help with that. And so, it turned out, did Howard's doctor.

He prescribed antidepressants for his emotional condition, and after the magical month of in-patient treatment, released Howard back to his family and the care of us in his AA group. Ten years, later he's still taking his anti-depressants and is still going to AA.

Go figure.

So, is he an alcoholic or a drug addict? I don't know; I never drank with him. He says he is an alcoholic, and that's all that is needed to be an AA member. He was my friend too, until he decided he could no longer confide in me because I no longer attend AA meetings and/or because I now drink socially.

I miss his friendship; it feels like he has died. We used to be close.

He is also as atypical as anyone I've ever met in AA—a classic success story of the modern AA and **treatment center** industry. And my continued criticism, after these many years is this:

The AA and **treatment center** approach to the drug and/or alcohol related problems we faced is "either/or" (meaning, either do it our way or get out). If you had any kind of problem with emotional issues and drug or alcohol abuse, then there is no other choice: "we have to treat you for alcoholism, and no, sorry, there just isn't any other way."

You will either become 1) a "victim of alcohol," an alcoholic, and therefore get the treatment you obviously need or 2) we, the AA-**treatment center** industry will only see you as just being hopeless, and you are out of luck or help in either case.

Or, as in the cancer hospital analogy I referred to earlier: treatment equals chemotherapy, sort of.

I have met many such fellow sufferers over the years who AA has helped. These were people who were probably not alcoholic but were told, nonetheless, that since they met some sort of **treatment center** diagnosis as being a chemically dependent person, they could then join AA and participate in its meetings.

It might also be that unspoken secret everybody knows about, which is *if you feel that AA meetings alone aren't meeting your needs, do not despair; we have drugs to help you.* Please do not confuse this with the timeworn problem of depressed AA members self-medicating, for example.

Self-medication is discouraged for obvious reasons. Unless, of course, you are on a doctor's prescription for antidepressants. Lots of AA members are on antidepressants. In my opinion, this has become the social lubricant of AA, a new and approved substitute for the coffee/nicotine/sugar combo most of the original and early members of AA used so effectively to calm down while also stimulating conversation in the meeting rooms.

Practically everyone says these new drugs are needed for their recovery. How did early AA ever get along without all this medicine? Not very well, evidently.

Chapter 20
Where Did This Train Go "Off the Tracks"?

In my humble opinion, which seems to be supported by the research I've done, AA's recovery success is at about 5 to 10 percent. Not nearly the foolproof success they imply in the beginning of their meetings with the reading of chapter 5 of the Big Book: "Rarely have we seen a person fail who has thoroughly followed our path. Those who do not recover are people who cannot or will not completely give themselves to this simple program, usually men and women who are constitutionally incapable of being honest with themselves!"[1]

If one reads this passage carefully, isn't AA calling the unfortunate and skeptical ones who *do not* buy this program hook, line, and sinker delusional—or worse—liars?

I guess they are, for this passage goes on like this: "There are such unfortunates. They are not at fault; they seem to have been born that way. They are naturally incapable of grasping and developing a manner of living which demands rigorous honesty."

Again, AA's allegation that the alcoholic's problem lies in the fact that he is dishonest (which he probably is). They go on: "Their chances are less than average. There are those, too, who suffer from grave emotional and mental disorders, but many of them do recover if they have the capacity to be honest."

You may not agree with my logic here, and that is OK with me, but the key point that I am making about the entire concept of AA is this:

The recovery of the alcoholic (or "chemically dependent") individual hinges on him or her grasping the way of life of one who has "thoroughly followed our [their] path."

I know this firsthand because I too did this successfully for over thirty years. I was among the *true believers* in AA who buy the concept of it as a way of recovery. Those who do not are out of luck. There is nothing wrong with this "way of life" approach, unless you happen to not agree with it.

There has accumulated an encyclopedic amount of statistics about AA. These statistics and voluminous research support the complaints I have made in this chapter and elsewhere in this book: namely that while AA is a religion and a lifestyle guide, it is **NOT** a cure for anything.

In a *Wikipedia* search of the term *AA recovery* I found, (among others) that Dr. Lance Dodes, former director of substance abuse treatment at Harvard's McLean Hospital and assistant clinical professor of psychiatry at Harvard Medical School, says Alcoholics Anonymous helps between 5 percent and 10 percent of its participants. Dodes also believes AA harms **90** percent of participants because of the perception that "If you fail in AA, it's you that's failed" and not AA.[2]

What is happening at AA meetings generally is this: a group of people who have had a collective experience about abstaining from drinking, on which they all agree, meet and discuss the talking points of the twelve steps at their meetings.

This research uncovered that *the key point* is this: AA doesn't magically make people stop drinking alcohol or doing mood-altering drugs.

These folks had already decided *on their own* that they had to stop their substance abuse, which some us of call a behavior as opposed to an addiction. This is why they decide to and are able to quit!

They continue to go to AA to be with like-minded individuals to share the experience with and support each other in this effort.

There is nothing wrong with this activity other than what they tell the approximately 90 percent of people who try AA, find it seriously lacking for themselves, and therefore do not buy into this *simple program* that AA claims to offer. That is, they are considered to be both mentally defective and morally dishonest because AA doesn't work for them!

What a message to leave with an already-suffering person.

Contrary to the chapter 5 text on how it works, there are millions of former alcohol and drug abusers out there who neither go to meetings nor endorse the concepts of AA and are doing very well with their lives. Some of them—and I have met many—have returned to social and responsible drinking, too. That includes me—for more than three years.

In another posting Dr.Dodes made the following comment, that the vast majority of the people who successfully quit drinking for a year or more, 80% of them, "do it alone, all by themselves, without any treatment program or support group."

Another study reported in the *Harvard Mental Health Letter* of October 1995 found that 80 percent of all alcoholics who recover for a year or more do so on their own, some after being successfully treated. When a group of these self-treated alcoholics was interviewed, 57 percent said they simply decided that alcohol was bad for them, and 29 percent said health problems, frightening experiences, accidents, or blackouts persuaded them to quit. Others used such phrases as "things were building up" or "I was sick and tired of it." According to researchers, "Support from a husband or wife was important in sustaining the resolution."[1]

Naturally, those do-it-yourselfers will also insist they have a surefire solution that really works:
"Just don't drink any more alcohol, ever (if necessary)!"

I know that many of my former fellow AA members turn a blind eye to such simple logic. An anecdote (not antidote) illustrating the folly of not recognizing this logic follows:
A bunch of people went to a Baptist church for years.

During these years, many of the women got pregnant and had babies.

This proves going to Baptist churches causes women to get pregnant.

This is the same goofy logic that AA uses to "prove" that because people go to AA meetings, they stay sober.

- AA chooses not to see or care that these members go to AA meetings because they want to "stay quit" of drinking, not "to quit."
- It is not because the members have gone to meetings that they've quit.
- The reason that they finally did quit is this: *they were afraid of the consequences of their continued use of drugs and alcohol such as divorce, loss of jobs, death, etc.*

So much for the AA viewpoints: "Everybody needs a support group" and "Nobody can do it alone."

Actually, most successfully recovered people do it alone.

Chapter 21
Summary

I had spent half of my life in the twelve-step program of Alcoholics Anonymous. How did I just walk away from this and why?

To answer these questions, I remember, as AA teaches, "what we used to be like, what happened and what we are like now."[1] In my humble opinion, I am the poster child for ADD: attention deficit disorder.

I was as a child and still am as an adult.

My mother remarked recently, just before she passed away, that a wonderful nun I'd had in eighth grade, Sister Giovanni, commented to her at a parent/teacher meeting, "I just don't know what gets into that boy." Sister G. went on to establish a home for delinquent youth on the city's notorious South Side, many years later. I like to think that I had at least added to her inspiration to do so.

I wasn't a bad kid, just easily bored. And so I had run-ins with the police and other authorities; with parents of other children for fighting; and with local shop owners for stealing and vandalism. That was on top of the poor concentration I showed early on in the classroom. In general, it was just misspent youthful energy.

Another anecdote from my youth: One summer day when I was about fourteen or fifteen, Roger, Greg, and I found a small railroad utility cart chained near the railroad track spur near our neighborhood We quickly figured out how to break the chain and lock and free the little eight-foot-by-eight-foot cart. Using a small, sturdy tree branch as a fulcrum, we pried it up onto the tracks. Not seeing or hearing any trains coming near us, we decided to take this little cart for a joy ride, using the branch to push it along. We knew the direction we had taken, back toward the city, had a gradual downward grade.

Within minutes. we were moving along at a pace too rapid to encourage jumping off. Besides, the way seemed clear, and we were having a blast. Soon the cart was racing past city street intersections at the railroad crossings, and at each one, the crossing guards came down with ringing bells and flashing lights to stop the auto and truck traffic.

While we could see this taking place, we were powerless to stop it, nor did we want to. All these years later, I still sense the feeling of that wagon humming along and flying down the railroad tracks. The wind in my face, whipping my hair and clothes, felt wonderful. I felt like the captain of this runaway ship instead of being its captive.

Mile after mile, one crossing guard after another flashed by, stopping bewildered auto drivers, as we three juvenile vagabonds flew along on this unplanned joyride, precariously balancing ourselves with nothing to hang on to, just our own nimble footwork. No seats or safety belts on this thrill ride!

Soon we heard police sirens in our vicinity, and we knew it was only a matter of time before the ride and "the jig" was up. The cart finally slowed down near the old Hamm's beer brewery, after about ten miles. There were at least three or four squad cars and police waiting for us. Some of the cops were laughing. We three got to ride in the back seat of one of the squad cars to the St. Paul police station booking room. We were charged there for vandalism, theft, and other assorted offenses too numerous to detail.

The judge, with a barely suppressed smirk, released us to our parents' custody with the warning "If you boys are caught breaking the law in any way again, you will go to jail."

Our parents all promised we never would. And, good to our word, we were never caught again.

The rest of my story continues at the beginning of this book. The connection I am attempting to make is this: while I always had difficulty with my so-called self-control, I was also capable of achieving life successes too.

While always well intentioned, I often have difficulty in the area of follow-through. A life history of adventures, welcome and unwelcome, has been part of my legacy. What brought me to AA—that first meeting with Steve K. and subsequent times, thereafter—was a search for something to help me control my life. Religion and my nine years of Catholic school didn't do it; I'd finish the last three at a public high school.

The navy might have been just what I needed, if only I could have stayed in. Again, not my choice.

Both my first and subsequent attempts at AA membership were much more about me finding the things I deeply felt were missing from my life: control (as in some rules to guide me), purpose (for example, attempting to stay sober while helping others), and a group or a club that was unique enough to have or even want me as a member.

AA fulfilled all three of these needs for me. It became a place for me to achieve prominence for doing good works by helping others, which brought with it recognition and opportunity to do more and to meet connected people who wanted a man like me on their team (another first).

It was my way of life for over three decades. It was the glue that held my marriage to Susie together too.

Not surprisingly, I tried to leave AA many times over the years. I changed my meeting days, and when that didn't satisfy the angst I felt, I knew this AA recovery thing just wasn't relevant any more.

I had changed clubs and formats, even the parts of town where I attended meetings, just to find what I used to enjoy there: seeing new faces, doing anything that would help make my work there feel important again, like it used to.

I finally returned to the old North Oakdale club, and to the Wednesday meeting at 6:00 p.m., because that's where my ex-wife, Susie had gone, and she had made many friends there. She had gotten involved with volunteer service work, too, sponsoring new women members, and had been very well regarded there.

Until she too grew bored with it all.

Remember, Susie had attended AA about a year more than I had. When she left our marriage two years ago, it was the second time she had done so. She had also left me in that same month, August, one year earlier.

That time she was only gone for a couple of months, until she asked if I would take her back. What I didn't know was she had decided to stop attending AA, and as reported earlier, she had taken up social drinking during that time. This pretty much negated her AA membership too. She was fully aware of the consequences. No one had been a better student or trusted servant of Alcoholics Anonymous then she had been over the thirty-plus years she had attended.

She had become completely disillusioned with it all as well.

Today, more than three years since I quit AA and began this new way of life, I remain a dedicated social drinker, period. I have gone through the holidays, birthdays, a serious fall and broken bone, being broke for a time, and turning sixty-five years of age—all without the support of a wife of a steady job—and have not gotten drunk once, despite weathering these and other problems.

For a while, I did try a men's Al-Anon group along with a book-study group that researches Al-Anon teachings about how the so-called codependent partners of alcoholics live with alcoholism. After a several-month trial, it was very clear that this wasn't working either. Several old demons reared their heads:

First of all, the first step of Al-Anon is the same as in AA: "We admitted we were powerless over alcohol and that our lives had become unmanageable."

So are most of the other steps' terminologies: "powerlessness, out of control, insanity, finding recovery through God," etc.

I am no longer in any of those places. I was dealing with being an underemployed, over-sixty-five-year-old man who was about to have a single's life thrust upon him. I was sometimes frightened, saddened, angry, and feeling hopeless.

But since I am *not insane*, or anything like it, why the f**k—would I need to be "restored to sanity?"

"Where I believe AA Failed ME"

As I said, AA was the glue that held my marriage together (maybe for too damn long, it turns out). There were also other issues that I spoke of, such as the failure in my career and other related things. But, after all of the years I spent following the program, *to the letter*, AA ultimately did *almost nothing* to help solve these matters; in fact, quite *the opposite* became true.

Reliance upon AA, through my attendance at meetings, kept me from seeking the counseling I needed to solve these matters. This is a harsh claim to be sure, and certainly, a blaming one. But *blame* really begs to be discussed here.

As I said earlier, I did talk about my problems repeatedly in my AA meeting, to no avail. In addition, my continued attendance at these meetings, at this critical time in my life, both *stalled and distracted* me from getting the more personal help I desperately needed. Why bother?

I've come to believe that **AA is so thorough at keeping itself positioned as the "only recovery" vehicle any practicing** *true believer* **needs, you would have to be crazy to not believe it to be so.** But then sometimes, you do become crazy from the stress in your life.

Do you think that sounds harsh?

They constantly tell you this is so through the not-so-subtle text of the Big Book. Please follow along as I share with you the phrases a newcomer may only discern after countless meetings.

Here are some key points (often overlooked):

Step One: "…(that) we were powerless" and "…our lives had become unmanageable."

Step Two: "…a power greater than ourselves could restore us to sanity."

Step Three: "...to turn our will and our lives over to the care of God..." (And this isn't a religion?)

Step Four: "...made a searching and fearless moral inventory of ourselves."

Steps Five through Seven: (where we) "...admitted to God, 'ourselves and another person' the exact nature of our wrongs." (We were then ready to) "...have God remove all these defects of character," (and finally) "...asked him (God) to remove our shortcomings."

This inventory and restitution phase concludes somewhat with the so-called Fifth Step Prayer on page 76:

"When ready, we say something like this: 'My creator, I am now willing that you should have all of me, good and bad. I pray that you now remove from me every single defect of character which stands in the way of my usefulness to you and my fellows. Grant me strength as I go out from here, to do your bidding. Amen.'" **Powerful words to any true believer.**

But what if it doesn't work anymore?

The detritus that remained of my AA involvement only could offer me this advice: *you'll just have to keep doing it over and try harder this time!* Remember what they told us in chapter 5, page 58: "rarely have we seen a person fail who has *thoroughly* followed our (the) path."

These words may actually have an influence on you, for good or not, from the very beginning. I saw it happen over and over with new attendees. These were frequently sick people who needed to get control over their substance abuse *and* their lives. The solution that AA insinuates here? You are a. insane, b. crazy, and c. out-of-control, and therefore **only God can save you.**

Don't get me wrong; I am OK with this to a point, for some. I have seen newcomers who were at their last hope when they reached us. However, as I have said before, this thing known as *AA recovery* was not intended as a "mental health" tune-up, in my opinion. Neither is it a clinical approach to recovery. It is, instead, as they like to say in AA, a **"spiritual healing."** *I call it a fix.*

Well, isn't that like a religion?

After you have recovered and stayed sober for a long enough time, and, as AA suggests, you have worked with newcomers and kept on going to meetings, it all looks the same. Nothing really changes, except (and you do not notice this right away), many of the people you've gone to meetings with for years have stopped showing up!

Oh, they have been replaced by more newcomers over time, but not proportionately. The club's meeting groups may have grown somewhat (not always, though). Many of those who have stopped showing up are not replaced, and some AA clubs have had to close their doors (occasionally).

Observing further, if you are a member of an AA club that did expand, you may notice something: the expansion is **not in proportion** *to the numbers of new people who have joined, or the club would have outgrown its meeting rooms by now.*

Very few clubs have had that luxury lately.

Back to my crisis. At the time that Susie left me, I not only *wasn't getting help from AA* any longer, but it had become the *ultimate placebo (distraction)* —one that likely would have *killed me*—if I had not stopped trying to use "the program" soon enough.

Some will tell you that they were coached by a member in their AA squad to seek outside professional help. I've had occasion to offer this advice to men I was sponsoring. This is well and good too, *if it does take place*. This time, for me, it did not, no one suggested outside help for me.

Had I not been so overwhelmed with adversity from every corner, I might prescribed it for myself. This has since been corrected.

I did see a Psychologist weekly for my emotional needs. She was aware of my previous decades-long attendance at AA and confided to me *that I am not the first former AA member she has counseled who attended meetings for so long with less-than-encouraging results.*

Susie and I have divorced. She has been living with her steady boyfriend for over a year. We speak occasionally, settling our estate details. *I thank the powers that be* that we are finally apart. No blame here (not too much), but we had become toxic together; our relationship just was no longer fixable.

My family has gotten reacquainted with me and now, also, MJ. Having a drink with them when we get together socially is an effective icebreaker. Nobody gets drunk. My brothers and sister have become a real comfort to me, and, I hope, I to them as well. We seem to like each other again, a nice change.

Instead of attending weekly AA meetings.

I now go out swing dancing with MJ at least two times a week. There is an endless menu of steps and styles to master there, and I expect to be at it for as long as I'm able. It reminds me of the roller-rink skate-dancing I did as a youth. Getting out of the house for a purpose that includes fellowship and good music both motivates me, and, happily, keeps me fit.

I work out at a fitness center 3 – 4 times weekly. I visit with many elderly people and am thinking of getting back into regular volunteering (which I had done for decades).

On page 164 of the Big Book of Alcoholics Anonymous is an invocation that had become a favorite of mine. I thought of it again while I did the final edit of these pages:

> *Our book is meant to be suggestive only. We realize we know only a little. God will constantly disclose more to you and to us. Ask Him in your morning meditation what you can do each day for the man who is still sick. The answers will come, if your own house is in order. But obviously you cannot transmit something you haven't got. See to it that your relationship with Him is right, and great events will come to pass for you and countless others. This is the great fact for us.*
>
> *Abandon yourself to God as you understand God. Admit your faults to Him and to your fellows. Clear away the wreckage of your past. Give freely of what you find and join us. We shall be with you in the Fellowship of the Spirit, and you will surely meet some of us as you trudge the Road of Happy Destiny.*
>
> *May God bless you and keep you—until then.*

What If?

The biggest obstacle to my finishing this work was this worry: *What if* some recovering drunk/addict read these pages and decided to also give up on abstinence and then drink or use drugs to a tragic result for him- or herself or someone else?

The question haunted me for many months. This was much more than writer's block. It was a moral dilemma.

I finally came to terms with this perplexing quandary one day recently, when I recalled what happened to Bill, an old apartment building neighbor.

Bill and Donna lived two floors below us in the first apartment Susie and I had rented. He was the assistant manager, and we all soon became card-playing friends.

Over many games of Five Hundred, we learned each other's stories, the four of us. Bill had served prison time for a series of drunken-behavior crimes—driving drunk, drunk and-disorderly behavior, breaking and entering—all as a repeat felon going back to his youth.

As a felon, he was not allowed to own firearms. He had many, however: all bigger-bore .45s and 9mm Glock. He also had attended AA, going back more than twenty years, without achieving any continuous sobriety. I observed him in a less-than-sober condition on numerous occasions.

Donna was one of the sweetest women I have ever met. She and Bill had a daughter, Dawn, who mirrored her mom. Handsome, charming to a fault, with a wonderful sense of humor, Bill had everything to live and strive for. Donna adored him.

One morning, sometime after the bars closed at 1:00 a.m., Bill was arrested while staggering down the middle of a street in a poorer part of town. What brought attention from the residents and, therefore, the police, were his shouted epithets promising punishment to the effing cops for what they did to him, while brandishing a high-powered gun in each hand!

He now had a new resentment to add to his list; he was sent back to prison. Soon after, his wife died from a heart condition that Susie and I believe was also a broken heart. He had crushed the hope out of her. Dawn went to live with a favorite aunt.

Bill got drunk that night for his own reasons, and AA could not save him. I have no way of knowing if a plan such as mine could have made any difference to him or anyone like him.

Repeated attempts at "the program" certainly hadn't helped Bill. I had even sponsored him for a time and heard his Fifth step inventory. I certainly hadn't felt that I was witnessing a doomed man.

Twenty-five years later, I still feel sad about what happened to Bill and his family. AA says if you don't take the first drink, you cannot get drunk. What about the people who, for their own reasons, cannot choose to not take that first drink? I know of so many Bills out there who just keep failing at it. Is AA's complete-abstinence approach really the only solution for *all* of them?

So, I dedicate this last chapter to the memory of Bill, Donna, and Dawn.

Three years ago I said good by to John C., the other Howard C., Tom, Sue, Theresa, Gary, Pam, Lefty and all of the *true believers*. "Keep the lights burning guys".

I have a family that loves me, a beautiful woman who will soon be my wife, everything to live and achieve for, as long as I stick to my plan, my wine and beer diet. They all deserve at least that much from me, as we toast our lives together over a glass of *the beverage of our choice.*

Howard Casanova - howardcasanova@gmail.com

My Axioms

I still live a day at a time, even a moment at a time.

I try to practice moderation in all things.

I value my friends even more now; they have all become people I socialize with, but no longer do I attend AA meetings with any of them.

My family is my most valued treasure.

I seek the advice and counsel of both those who befriend me and those I need to seek out.

The program teaches, "We will not regret the past nor wish to shut the door on it,"[1] sage advice I still follow to keep the effects of my memories in check and to deal honorably with the uncomfortable ones.

I no longer really need a job to survive, but I need to feel useful, so I am looking into more satisfying work. Some nice options have appeared and will have my attention very soon.

I am still exploring my relationship with the *God of my understanding*, my higher power; I have never been much of a spiritual person, but I am quite an emotional one.

I still tend to isolate and fear the things I am threatened by, but I know that taking action is a great leveler. I may have to practice courage whenever I do feel fear, but I go ahead regardless.

When I was a child, I would hear TV's Davy Crockett say, "Be sure you're right, then go ahead." I still think of that a lot.

I also recollect a character named Eddie Haskel on *Leave it to Beaver*, who often said, "You look really nice today, Mrs. Cleaver" to Beaver's mom. Compliment the ladies, especially the ones who need a little help.

When I am faced with adversity, I respond as if challenged.

I try to be succinct; really, I do, all the time, even more sometimes.

The late comic W. C. Fields frequently advised, "Never give a sucker an even break." I'd guess that he didn't suffer fools well either.

I find that counseling myself not to panic, seek out disaster, feed my failure fears, or give in to anger produces very good results. I tell myself, "Calm down," "Everything is OK," "You're doing good," etc. I really do listen to myself!

My memory is much better than I had previously thought, but I challenge myself there, too. Playing cards on Monday evening, daily online Scrabble, Lumosity, and so on. I love to read: crime novels, travelogues—especially about long-distance sailing—biographies, news links to daily local and national stories, etc. Most recently I have read the autobiography of Bernard Moitessier.

After a lifetime of friction, I made peace with my aged ninety-three-year-old mother, well before she recently passed. Now I can cherish a heartfelt grieving of her loss, instead of harboring old resentments. Very freeing for me.

The less I acknowledge my tormenters, the taller I am able to stand.

When I'm tempted to lie, cheat, exaggerate, gossip, etc., I ask myself, "How's that integrity thing working out?"

I recommend having or doing something you can be passionate about. I have always been happiest when sailing, so MJ and I have recently acquired a thirty-seven-foot sailboat, S/V Unity, which we sail up on Lake Superior. More adventures await us there.

The greatest evidence of love is undying loyalty. When I told MJ that I loved her, I was saying that I have taken myself off of the market to other women. I am no longer shopping around.

The Beer/Wine Diet

"I'll have a side of water with that."

On any day I may imbibe, I keep the following in mind: one drink relaxes me, but if I drink more than one before one and a half to two hours have elapsed, I may end up feeling too intense.

So, two (beers or glasses of wine) in two to three hours is generally my limit. Rarely, a third beer or wine, and then only after an hour or more has passed since the second one!

I have successfully kept to this alcohol intake limit for more than three years.

I choose to not comment on the consumption of other alcoholic beverages, as I rarely indulge in any beyond an occasional sip.

Note: The secret is to always order a side of water with wine or beer! This way, you still have something to sip on for an hour or more after you have drunk the alcohol beverage.

You can always order more water, and food always helps!
HC

END NOTES

Introduction
    "Gimme Some Old-Time Religion…"..................8
Dr. Stanton Peele, 1998, *The Sciences, p.17 – 21,* [1]
Dr. Lance Dodes: *The Sober Truth: Debunking the Bad Science Behind 12-Step Programs and the Rehab Industry.*[2]
1983 *Cambridge Somerville Program for Alcohol Rehabilitation* (CASPAR) Study.[3]
October 1939, *Journal of the American Medical Association* (JAMA)[4]

Chapter 8
    When AA Changed Forever................................43
1990 National Longitudinal Alcohol Epidemiologic Survey (NLAES)[1]
Big Book, Chapter 3, p.30, para.1, sentence 4, thru 6.[2]

Chapter 9
    The AA Cure 49
Big Book, Chapter 5, p. 58, para.1.[1]
Big Book, Chapter 5, p. 59, step 3.[2]

Chapter 14
    Out the Back Door of AA 71
Big Book, Forward, p. xiii[1]
1983 *Cambridge Somerville Program for Alcohol Rehabilitation* (CASPAR) Study.[2]
Dr. Lance Dodes: *The Sober Truth: Debunking the Bad Science Behind 12-Step Programs and the Rehab Industry.*[3]
Big Book, p.*58, para. 3.*[4]

Chapter 15
    My Perfect Storm 80
http;//www.meetup.com[1]

Chapter 17
    Why Bother to Write This Book?......................93
    Big Book, Forward, p.xiii[1]

Chapter 18
    In Defense of AA, but also of the 90+ Percent Who Cannot, Will Not Fit-in There 95
    Dr. Lance Dodes: *The Sober Truth: Debunking the Bad Science Behind 12-Step Programs and the Rehab Industry.*[1]
    The Responsibility Pledge of Alcoholics Anonymous," introduced in July 1965 at the 30th Anniversary International Convention in Toronto, Canada.[2]
    Big Book, Chapter 5, p. 59, steps 4 & 5.[3]

Chapter 20
    Where Did This Train Go "Off the Tracks"? .104
    Big Book, Chapter 5, p. 58, para.1.[1]
    Dr. Lance Dodes: *The Sober Truth: Debunking the Bad Science Behind 12-Step Programs and the Rehab Industry.*[2]
    Treatment of Drug Abuse and Addiction—Part Three," *Harvard Mental Health Letter* 12, no 4 (October 1995): 3.

Chapter 21
    Summary..109
    Big Book, Chapter 5, p. 58, para.2.[1]

My Axioms 119
    Big Book, Chapter 6, p. 83, para.4.[1]

Made in the USA
San Bernardino, CA
11 January 2017